GENETICS – RESEARCH AND ISSUES

DISCRETE OPTIMIZATION FOR TSP-LIKE GENOME MAPPING PROBLEMS

GENETICS – RESEARCH AND ISSUES

GENETICS – RESEARCH AND ISSUES

DISCRETE OPTIMIZATION FOR TSP-LIKE GENOME MAPPING PROBLEMS

D. MESTER
D. RONIN
M. FRENKEL
A. KOROL
Z. BRÄYSY
O. DULLAERT
AND
W. RAA

Nova Science Publishers, Inc.
New York

For permission to use material from this book please contact us:
Telephone 631-231-7269; Fax 631-231-8175
Web Site: http://www.novapublishers.com

NOTICE TO THE READER

LIBRARY OF CONGRESS CATALOGING-IN-PUBLICATION DATA

Discrete optimization for TSP-like genome mapping problems / D. Mester ...
[et al.].
    p. ; cm.
  Other title: Discrete optimization for traveling salesperson problem-like
genome mapping problems
  Includes bibliographical references and index.
  ISBN 978-1-61668-170-8 (softcover)
  1. Gene mapping--Mathematical models. 2. Mathematical optimization. I.
Mester, D. (David) II. Title: Discrete optimization for traveling
salesperson problem-like genome mapping problems.
  [DNLM: 1. Chromosome Mapping--methods. 2. Algorithms. QU 450 D611 2010]
  QH445.2.D57 2010
  572.8'633--dc22

                                                    2010001744

Published by Nova Science Publishers, Inc. ✦ New York

CONTENTS

PREFACE

Several problems in modern genome mapping analysis belong to the field of discrete optimization on a set of all possible orders. Here we describe formulations, mathematical models and algorithms for genetic/genomic mapping problem, that can be presented in TSP-like terms. These include: ordering of marker loci (or genes) in multilocus genetic mapping (MGM), multilocus consensus mapping (MCGM), and physical mapping problem (PMP). All these problems are considered as computationally challenging because of noisy marker scores, large-size data sets, specific constraints on certain classes of orders, and other complications. The presence of specific constrains on ordering of some elements in these problems does not allow applying effectively the well-known powerful discrete optimization algorithms like Cutting-plane, Genetic algorithm with EAX crossover and famous Lin-Kernighan. In the paper we demonstrate that developed by us Guided Evolution Strategy algorithms successfully solves this class of discrete constrained optimization problems. The efficiency of the proposed algorithm is demonstrated on standard TSP problems and on three genetic/genomic problems with up to 2,500 points.

Chapter 1

1. GENERAL INTRODUCTION

Several computationally challenging problems related to genetic (genomic) analysis belong to the field of discrete optimization on a set of all possible orders. In particular, genetic and genomic problems that can be formulated in such terms include: ordering of marker loci (or genes) in multilocus genetic mapping (*MGM*), multilocus consensus genetic mapping (*MCGM*) and physical mapping problem (*PMP*). Different elements can be ordered in these problems, including genes, DNA markers, DNA clones.

The essence of multipoint genome mapping problems is unravel the linear order of the elements (genes, DNA markers, or clones) based on the measured matrix of pairwise distances d_{ij} between these elements. With n elements the number of the possible orders is $n!/2$ out of which only one is considered as a true order. A primary difficulty in ordering genomic elements is the large number of possible orders. In real problems, n might vary from dozens to thousands and more. Exact solution to the problem that can be obtained on 3000 Mhz modern computer is $n=14$ after one hour. Clearly, already with $n>15$ it would not be feasible to evaluate all $n!/2$ possible orders using two-point linkage data. In addition to the large number of possible order, the mapping problems are difficult for solving because of noisy marker scores, large-size data sets, specific constraints on certain classes of orders, and other complications.

Historically, the main approach of ordering markers within linkage groups to produce genetic maps was based on multipoint maximum likelihood analysis. Several effective algorithms have been proposed using various optimization tools, including branch and bound method (Lathrop *et al.*, 1985), simulated annealing (Thompson, 1984; Weeks and Lange, 1987; Stam, 1993;

Jansen *et al.*, 2001), and seriation (Buetow and Chakravarti, 1987). Computational complexity does not allow applying this approach for large scale problems.

Olson and Boehnke (1990) compared eight different methods for marker ordering. In addition to multilocus likelihood, they also considered more simple criteria for multipoint marker ordering in large-scale problems based on two-point linkage data (by minimizing the sum of adjacent recombination rates or adjacent genetic distances). The simple criteria are founded on the biologically reasonable assumption that the true order of a set of linked loci will be the one that minimizes the total map length of the chromosome segment. As an alternative to maximum likelihood multilocus analysis, multipoint ordering problem can be addressed by using the methods and algorithms developed for the classical formulation of Traveling Salesperson Problem (TSP) (Press *et al.*, 1986; Week and Lange, 1987; Falk, 1992; Schiex and Gaspin, 1997). Here we consider three groups of genome mapping problems that can be efficiently solved based on heuristics developed for TSP: multilocus genetic mapping (*MGM*), multilocus consensus mapping (*MCGM*) and physical mapping problem (*PMP*).

MGM can be reduced to a particular case of TSP referred to as Wandered Salesperson Problem (WSP). In fact, the genomic ordering problems are "uni-dimensional" WSP (UWSP) because all elements belong to one coordinate axis only in accordance with the basic organization of genetic material in the chromosomes. WSP is a particular case of the TSP in which the salesperson can start wherever he/she wishes and does not have to return to the starting city after visiting all cities (Papadimitiou and Steiglitz, 1981). In contrast to classical TSP, UWSP formulation reflects the real fact that the genetic maps of all eukaryotic organisms have a beginning and end points. Moreover, genetic/genomic problems reduced formally to TSP have some specified particularities and complications: *(a)* before construction of the maps we must divide the datasets of markers (or clones in physical mapping) into non-overlapping sets corresponding to chromosomes and linkage groups (or contigs of clones); this step can be referred to as *clustering stage*; *(b)* some points of the solution may have known (predefined) order (*anchor markers*); *(c)* the genetic or physical distance between two points on a chromosome, d_{ij}, can not be measured exactly due to noises in scoring and other complications. Because of these complications, the *true ordering* of the points may not provide the optimum value of the optimization criterion (minimal total distance). By this reason, to unravel the true order we must verify the stability of the solution with respect to stochastic variation of the distance matrix.

For solving the TSP, several well-known heuristic algorithms can be applied: Tabu Search (TS), Simulated Annealing (SA), Guided Local Search (GLS), Genetic Algorithm (GA), Evolution Strategy (ES), Guided Evolution Strategy (GES), Ant Colony Behavior (ACB), Artificial Neural Networks (ANN), and Cutting-plane (for detailed references see Mester *et al.*, 2004). The presence of specific constrains on ordering of some elements in MGM does not allow applying effectively the well-known powerful discrete optimization algorithms like Cutting-plane (Chvatal *et al.*, 1999), GA with EAX crossover (Nagata and Kobayashi, 1997; Nagata, 2007), and LandK (Helsgaun, 2000; Applegate *et al.*, 2003).

MCGM is a further considerable complication of genome mapping problem caused by the need of combining the mapping results from different labs. Two approaches were suggested to solve *MCGM* problems, both looking for shared orders with maximum number of shared markers. The first is based on "giving credit" to the available maps. To obtain the consensus solution, it employs different heuristics, e.g., graph-analytical method based on voting over median partial orders (Jackson *et al.*, 2007). The second approach is based on two-phase algorithm that on *Phase I* performs multilocus ordering combined with iterative re-sampling to evaluate the stability of marker orders. On this phase, the problem is reduced to TSP. Powerful metaheuristic, referred to as *GES*, can be applied to solve TSP (Mester *et al.*, 2004).

On *Phase II,* we consider consensus mapping as a new variant of TSP that can be formulated as *synchronized-TSP* (sTSP), and MCGM is solved by minimizing the criterion of weighted sum of recombination lengths along all multilocus maps. For the considered mapping problem we developed a new version of *GES* algorithm which defines consensus order for all shared markers (Mester *et al.*, 2005; Korol *et al.*, 2009). This approach is extended in chapter 2.

PMP is a genomic problem that also includes multipoint ordering to be addressed by reduction to TSP. The essence of PMP is assembling contigs from overlapping DNA clones using marker data and fingerprinting information (reviewed in Marra *et al.*, 1999). The true order of clones will be the one that minimizes the total number of gaps. Main complications in solving PMP are the large number of clones in cluster (with $n \sim 100\text{-}500$), noisy data and the possibility for similarity of non-adjacent clones due to abundance of repeated DNA in the genomes of higher eukaryotes (Lander *et al.*, 2001; Coe *et al.*, 2002; Gregory *et al.*, 2002; Faris and Gill, 2002). We developed a new effective method of clustering and contig ordering based on global optimization assisted by re-sampling verification process (analogously to Mester *et al.*, 2003a). Consequently, longer contigs can be obtained compared to the ordering results based on local optimization methods (e.g., those implemented in the standard FPC software Soderlund *et al.*, 2000).

Genomic applications described in this paper are based on our powerful Guided Evolution Strategy (GES) algorithms that combine two heuristics: Guided Local Search (GLS) (Voudouris, 1997; Tsang and Voudouris, 1997) and Evolution Strategy (Mester *et al.*, 2003a, 2004). Recently we developed and successfully tested some GES algorithms for more challenging discrete optimization problems known as Vehicle Routing Problems (Mester and Braysy, 2005; Mester and Braysy, 2006).

ES stage in GES algorithms is presented as a random search of optimum genotype of parameters by asexual reproduction, which uses *mutation*-derived variation and *selection*. The mutation changes of the current vector of parameters can be introduced by adding a vector of normally distributed variables with zero means. The level of changes can be defined by variances of these disturbances. Selection is another important stage of any ES algorithm. In GES algorithms we use (1+1) evolution strategies (Rechenberg, 1973) in which after each mutation the best solution vector is selected. During the optimization of the objective function, all mutations are performed on the best solution vector.

In the sections below we consequently show applications and adaptation of GES algorithm to solve standard TSP and three genetic/genomic problems.

2. GUIDED EVOLUTION STRATEGY ALGORITHM FOR CLASSIC TSP AS A BASIS FOR SOLVING THE GENETIC/GENOMIC TSP-LIKE PROBLEMS

2.1. INTRODUCTION

In this chapter we present the basic variant of GES metaheuristic for the classical symmetric TSP. This simple version of GES algorithm is referred to as Guided Local Search with Small Mutation (GLS-SM).

The TSP is one of the most basic, most important, and most investigated problems in combinatorial optimization. It consists of finding the cheapest tour (minimum total distance or some other cost measure associated with the performed trajectory) to sequentially visit a set of clients (cities, locations) starting and ending at the same client. We focus on the undirected (symmetric) TSP. The undirected TSP can be defined as follows. Let $G=(V, A)$ be a graph where $V=\{v_1,\ldots,v_n\}$ is the vertex set and $A=\{(v_i, v_j)|\ v_i, v_j \in V,\ i{\neq}j\}$ is an edge set, with a non-negative distance (or cost) matrix $C=(c_{ij})$ associated with A. The problem's resolution consists in determining the minimum cost Hamiltonian cycle on the problem graph. The symmetry is implied by the use of undirected edges (i.e., $c_{ij}{=}c_{ji}$). In addition, it is assumed that the distance matrix satisfies the triangle inequality ($c_{ij}{+}c_{jk}{>}c_{ik}$).

The TSP is known to be a NP-hard combinatorial optimization problem, implying that there is no algorithm capable of solving all problem instances in polynomial time. Heuristics are often the only feasible alternative to provide high-quality but not necessarily optimal solutions.

The TSP's apparent simplicity but intrinsic difficulty in finding the optimal solution has resulted in hundreds of publications. For excellent surveys, we refer to (Lawler et al., 1985; Reinelt, 1994; Burkard et al., 1998; Johnson and MCGeoch, 2002). Descriptions of the most successful and recent algorithms can be found in (Renaud et al., 1996; Tsang and Voudouris, 1997; Chvatal et al., 1999; Helsgaun, 2000; Applegate et al., 2003; Fisher and Merz, 2004; Walshaw, 2002; Schneider, 2003; Tsai et al., 2004; Cowling and Keuthen; 2005, Gamboa et al., 2006). There are also numerous industrial applications of TSP and its variants, varying from problems in transport and logistics (Lawler et al., 1985) to different problems in scheduling (Tsang and Voudouris, 1997; Pekney and Miller, 1991; Cowling, 1995), genetics (Mester et al., 2003a; Mester et al., 2003b; Mester et al., 2004; Mester et al., 2005) and electronics (Lin and Chen, 1996).

The main contribution of this chapter is developing a simple and efficient GLS-SM metaheuristic and demonstrating its performance on standard TSP benchmarks. The suggested metaheuristic combines the strengths of the well-known GLS metaheuristic (Voudouris, 1997) with a simple mutation phase to further facilitate escape from the local minimum. The mutation phase is based on the principles of evolution strategies (Rechenberg, 1973; Schwefel, 1977) and the 1-interchange improvement heuristic (Osman, 1993). In addition, we suggest a strategy for automatic tuning of the optimization parameters. The experimental tests on the standard TSP benchmarks demonstrate that the proposed algorithm is efficient and competitive with state-of-the-art algorithms.

The chapter is structured as follows. In the next part we describe the suggested metaheuristic, whereas section 2.3 details the algorithm configurations, experimental test setting and analysis of the computational results. Finally, in Section 2.4 conclusions are drawn.

2.2. THE PROBLEM SOLVING METHODOLOGY

The guided local search with small mutations (GLS-SM) metaheuristic starts with an initial solution in such that cities are listed in ascending order according to their sequence number in the input data. Then, a modified 2-opt improvement heuristic (Flood, 1956), described in the next subsection, is optionally applied to the solution before starting the metaheuristic search. The metaheuristic search is based on guided evolution strategies (Mester *et al.*, 2004) and active guided evolution strategies metaheuristics (Mester and Braysy, 2005; Mester and Braysy, 2006). It consists of two phases. The first phase makes use of the GLS metaheuristic as an aid to escaping local minima by augmenting the objective function with a penalty term based on particular solution features (e.g. long arcs) not considered to be part of a near-optimal solution. Here the GLS is used to guide a modified version of the classical 2-opt improvement heuristic, described in the next subsection. When no more improvements have been found for a given number of iterations, the second phase is started. In the second phase the GLS-SM further attempts to find an improved solution by performing a series of random 1-interchange moves, followed by local optimization with the modified 2-opt heuristic. As the possible improvement is checked only after 2-opt and because the number and type of modifications done each time are random, the second phase follows the principles of the (1+1)-evolution strategies metaheuristic. The second phase is repeated until no more improvements can be found. The search then goes back to the first phase, iterating repeatedly between both phases. The search is stopped by the user if no more improvements can be found in neither phases.

2.2.1. The Improvement Heuristics

Before proceeding to the detailed description of the suggested metaheuristic, we first describe the main features of the two improvement heuristics applied within our solution method. The standard 2-opt heuristic works by replacing two edges in the current solution by two other edges and iterates until no further improvement is possible. Figure 2.1 illustrates the 2-opt operator.

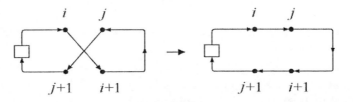

Figure 2.1 2-opt exchange operator. The edges $(i, i+1)$ and $(j, j+1)$ are replaced by edges (i, j) and $(i+1, j+1)$, thus reversing the direction of customers between $i+1$ and j.

To speed up the search, we suggest two variants of the standard 2-opt heuristic. Both variants work only on a limited neighborhood (except in the construction of the initial solution), denoted penalty variable neighborhood (PVN), detailed in the next subsection. The first variant, referred to as flexible 2-opt, adjusts the size of the PVN dynamically according to the possible improvements found. To be more precise, each time an improving move is found, the PVN is extended by four additional points, related to the end points l and m of the second exchanged edge that is located lower down in the current tour (j and $j+1$ in Figure 2.1). The goal of this extension is to perturb the search. Therefore, the algorithm selects the points l-1, l+1, m-1 and m+1 that are next to the indexes of l and m in the original problem data, provided that they are not already included in the PVN. After the improving move, the 2-opt is restarted using the extended PVN. The second variant, referred to as fast 2-opt, does not modify the PVN and it does not restart the search after improving moves. According to our experiments, fast 2-opt is 10–100 times faster than the flexible 2-opt but it results in lower solution quality as illustrated in Table 2.1 in section 2.3. This disadvantage of fast 2-opt is partially compensated by the next PVNs since the PVNs could be partially overlapped during the optimization process.

The fast and flexible 2-opt operators are applied here with the first-accept strategy, i.e., the solution information is updated right after each improving move. The 1-interchange was originally proposed for inter-route improvements in vehicle routing problems but here it is applied within a single TSP route. The idea is to swap simultaneously the position of two customers in the current tour. As described above, here the 1-interchange is applied together with a 2-opt variant and the possible improvement is checked only at the end after the 2-opt. In addition, only a limited set of random 1-interchange moves is considered.

2.2.2. Phase 1: A Guided Local Search Metaheuristic for the TSP

The GLS-SM metaheuristic consists of two phases: a GLS phase and a mutation phase. In the first phase a standard GLS metaheuristic is combined with either the flexible or the fast 2-opt variant. The GLS works by penalizing a single edge only every time the algorithm gets stuck in a local minimum. The edge chosen for penalization is the edge in the current solution for which the highest value of the following utility function is achieved by $U=c_{ij}^{*}/(1+p_{ij})$, where p_{ij} is the penalty counter for edge (i, j) which holds the number of times the edge has been penalized so far. The variable c_{ij}^* refers to the (virtual) penalized cost of the edges during the evaluation of the moves in the local search. It is only actually imposed for the arc with the highest utility value. This cost is calculated as $c_{ij}^* = c_{ij} + \lambda p_{ij}$, where c_{ij} refers to the original distances of the edges and $\lambda = \alpha L$ is a dynamic coefficient for determining the (virtual) penalized cost of an edge. Here α is a parameter and $L = \sum c_{ij}/n$ is the average length of the edges in the current (in the first phase) or in the current best (in the second phase) solution. By basing L and thus the penalties on the current and current best solution, it becomes possible to take into account the solution improvement during the search. This makes it possible to avoid penalty coefficients that are too high, which would otherwise allow the solution to deteriorate too much during the search. To diversify the search, the currently penalized edge is selected randomly with probability 0.001.

A new penalized edge is chosen every time when an improving move is found and at the beginning of both phases. In order to avoid calculating the penalized distances c_{ij}^* several times, they are stored in a matrix. After determining the edge to be penalized, the next step is to define the PVN that is used to restrict the local search to the neighborhood of the currently penalized edge (i, j). The forming of the PVN is illustrated at Figure 2.2.

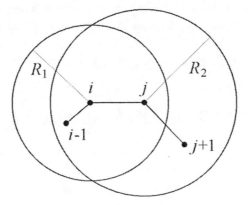

Figure 2.2. Illustration of creation the PVN. Here (i, j) is currently penalized edge , and two radiuses $R_1 = c_{ij} + c_{i-1,i}$ and $R_2 = c_{ij} + c_{j,j+1}$ define the size of PVN.

Based on the currently penalized edge (i, j), two radiuses $R_1 = c_{ij} + c_{i-1,i}$ and $R_2 = c_{ij} + c_{j,j+1}$ are calculated. Now all points of the problem within either R_1 or R_2 belong to the current PVN. Given that the PVN depends on the currently penalized edge and its neighboring edges, the size of the PVN is varying dynamically during the search. The old PVN is erased and a new PVN is defined at the beginning of each phase and also if an improvement is found. If the number of non-improving iterations c^1 exceeds a user-defined maximum, c^1_{max} , and if the PVN includes at least k points, the second phase is started.

2.2.3. Phase 2: Attempting Small Mutations

At the beginning of the second phase both the penalty edge and the PVN are redefined, as described above. Then, an attempt to improve the solution is made by performing r 1-interchanges randomly within the PVN followed by the local optimization of the obtained solution with either 2-opt variant. The number of moves, calculated as $r=3+22\xi^2$, where ξ is a random value uniformly distributed between 0 and 1. As opposed to the first phase, in the second phase the improvements are evaluated using the original distance matrix, instead of the GLS-based augmented objective function. In doing so, direct or real improvements to the objective function are evaluated after the mutation and selection processes. Local search within the second phase is continued until no more improvements can be found. In case improvements have been found in at least one of the two phases of the previous iteration of the GLS-SM, the search goes back to the first phase. Otherwise, the search is terminated. As deterioration is allowed, the algorithm maintains in memory the best solution found during the entire search and returns that solution at the end.

2.3. EXPERIMENTAL RESULTS

In this section we first describe the used parameter configurations as well as the problem data and the test environment used. Then, the results of computational testing on the suggested algorithm are presented, followed by a comparative analysis with state-of-art methods from the literature.

2.3.1. The Problem Data and Parameter Setting

The GLS-SM algorithm includes only three optimization parameters: the minimum number of points in the PVN to launch phase 2 (k), the weighting parameter α for setting the dynamic coefficient λ determining the (virtual) penalized cost of an edge and the maximum number of non-improving iterations of the first phase, c_{max}^1. In addition one can define whether or not fast 2-opt is applied in the creation for getting the initial solution and which of the proposed two 2-opt variants is used within the metaheuristic. We experimented with detailed tuning of these parameters for each test problem individually and we also tested a strategy for automatic tuning of these parameters. The detailed parameter values and the results are presented in Table 2.1. The value of parameter k is set to $k=10$ in all cases.

The following strategy, based on the information obtained during the individual tuning of the parameters, is used for the automatic tuning. For the construction of the initial solution and for the local search, only the fast 2-opt variant is applied. At the beginning c_{max}^1 is set to $c_{max}^1 = 2000$ and $\alpha=0.9$. Each time when $c^1 = 1000$, the value of α is decreased by 10%, c_{max}^1 is set to $c_{max}^1 = 200$ and c^1 is initialized to $c^1=0$. Correspondingly after each improving move c_{max}^1 is set to $c_{max}^1 = 2000$ and c^1 is set to $c^1 = 0$. In case α reaches value 0.2, the value of α is fixed to $\alpha=0.2$ and $c_{max}^1 =200$ is used during the rest of the search. Each time the parameter setting is changed, the penalty counters p_{ij} are reinitialized to zero.

The proposed GLS-SM metaheuristic has been implemented in Visual Basic 6.0 and the algorithm was executed on a Pentium IV Net Vista PC2800 MHz (512 Mb RAM) computer. The computational tests were carried out on 43 Euclidean symmetric TSP benchmarks (with 51–2392 points) taken from the TSPLIB (Reinelt, 1991) library. The selected problems are detailed in Table 2.1. The other problems from TSPLIB were not considered because the current implementation of the GLS-SM can only handle integer customer coordinates.

2.3.2. Analysis of Different Algorithm Configurations

In Table 2.1 we provide a comparative analysis of different algorithm configurations. The first column to the left lists the tested 43 problems with integer datasets. The numbers under problem name indicate the problem size. The second column gives the known optimal solution value (total distance) to each problem. The rest of the table is divided in two parts. In both parts we present the CPU time in seconds and perceptual excess with respect to the optimal solution. In the first part we examine the results obtained with automatic parameter tuning and compare results obtained only during the first phase of the algorithm (GLS) with the results of the whole algorithm (GLS-SM). In the second part we list the values used for individually optimized parameters α and c^1_{max} . For the parameter optimization, the following values were tested for α: 0.05, 0.1, 0.2, 0.25, 0.3, 0.35 and 0.4 and c^1_{max} : 20, 50, 100, 200, 250, 500, 1000, 2500 and 5000.

The sensitivity of the results with respect to parameter α is illustrated in Figure 2.3. According to the figure, there are quite significant differences in the results obtained with different values of α. Value $\alpha=0.2$ and values close to that seem to provide the best results. These values were therefore used in most of the experiments.

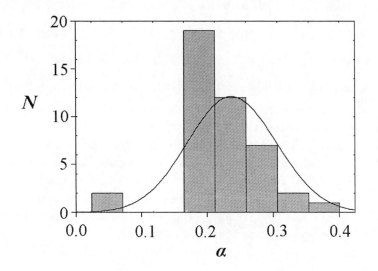

Figure 2.3 Distribution of the parameter α. The vertical axis represents the number of problems to which an optimal solution was found with the corresponding value of α (horizontal axis).

Figure 2.4 illustrates the sensitivity of the results with respect to parameter c^1_{max} . Again, it seems to be important to select a good parameter value. None of the parameter values can provide the optimal solution for all test problems, but in general a value of 20 seems to be the best. On the other hand, in several problems, very high values of c^1_{max} , close to 5000 appear to work well.

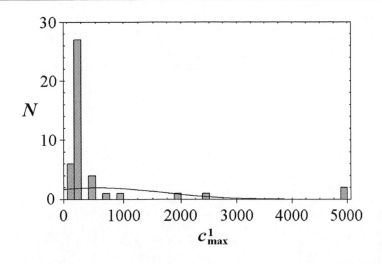

Figure 2.4. Distribution of the parameter c_{max}^1. As in Figure 2.3, the vertical axis describes the number of optimal solutions obtained with each parameter value.

In addition, for certain individual problems, some other exceptional values were attempted as well, as can be seen from Table 2.1. The results in the first set are obtained without applying 2-opt in the construction of the initial solution (poorer starting point for the metaheuristic) whereas in the second set 2-opt is used to provide higher quality initial solutions. The two sets differ also in the fact that in the first set fast 2-opt variant was applied and in the second set the flexible 2-opt operator.

In general, it appears from Table 2.1 that the results obtained by the GLS-SM metaheuristic are very close to the optimal. With the optimal parameter adjusting and usage of 2-opt in the initial solution construction, we obtained the optimal solution to all problems. The CPU times also seem to be reasonable, although for larger scale problems the required CPU time increases significantly. By comparing the first and second part, it can be observed that the results obtained with the automatic parameter tuning are only slightly worse than the results of optimized parameter values. It is interesting to note that in terms of CPU time the automatic tuning is faster. From the first part of Table 2.1 one can see that the GLS-SM algorithm gives both better and faster than average results, compared to the first GLS phase only. Based on the second part, it appears that better results can be obtained if a higher-quality initial solution is created with 2-opt and if the flexible 2-opt is applied. The differences are however small, in terms of both CPU time and solution quality, indicating the robustness of the procedures.

Table 2.1. Comparison of different algorithm configurations

Problem	Optimal	Self-tuning				Optimized parameters GLS-SM							
		GLS		GLS-SM		No 2-opt in initial solution				2-opt in initial solution			
		CPU	%	CPU	%	α	c^1_{max}	CPU	%	α	c^1_{max}	CPU	%
a280	2579	14.00	0	2.90	0	0.2	20	0.40	0	0.3	200	1.90	0
berlin52	7542	0.02	0	0.01	0	0.2	200	0.03	0	0.2	200	0.01	0
bier127	118282	14.00	0	2.80	0	0.2	200	0.31	0	0.25	200	0.40	0
eil51	426	1.30	0	0.06	0	0.2	200	0.06	0	0.3	250	0.06	0
eil76	538	0.05	0	0.06	0	0.3	200	0.06	0	0.2	250	0.05	0
eil101	629	0.10	0	0.30	0	0.3	200	0.12	0	0.2	250	0.10	0
kroA100	21282	0.08	0	0.30	0	0.2	200	0.06	0	0.2	200	0.10	0
kroB100	22141	0.05	0	0.35	0	0.3	200	0.12	0	0.25	200	0.10	0
kroC100	20749	0.05	0	0.06	0	0.3	200	0.06	0	0.25	200	0.10	0
kroD100	21294	3.50	0	0.06	0	0.2	200	0.06	0	0.25	200	0.10	0
kroE100	22068	2.50	0	2.90	0	0.3	200	0.12	0	0.25	200	0.20	0
kroA150	26524	1.98	0	2.20	0	0.2	100	0.40	0	0.2	200	0.30	0
kroB150	26130	0.05	0	1.60	0	0.2	200	0.18	0	0.2	200	0.30	0
kroA200	29368	11.00	0	3.50	0	0.2	200	0.30	0	0.2	200	0.67	0
kroB200	29437	5.50	0	1.60	0	0.2	200	0.50	0	0.25	200	0.58	0
lin105	14379	0.06	0	0.30	0	0.2	200	0.10	0	0.25	200	0.08	0
Linhp318	41345	14.00	0	4.96	0	0.3	200	1.20	0	0.3	2500	1.40	0
nrw1379	56638	187.00	0.26	126.00	0.04	0.25	500	260.00	0.04	0.25	2000	309.00	0
pcb442	50778	26.00	0	27.00	0.03	0.35	250	3.80	0	0.25	500	3.20	0

Problem	Optimal	Self-tuning				Optimized parameters GLS-SM							
		GLS		GLS-SM		No 2-opt in initial solution				2-opt in initial solution			
		CPU	%	CPU	%	α	c^1_{max}	CPU	%	α	c^1_{max}	CPU	%
pr76	108159	0.06	0	1.40	0	0.35	25	0.12	0	0.2	20	0.40	0
pr107	44303	5.10	0	0.68	0	0.2	200	0.30	0	0.2	200	0.67	0
pr124	59030	0.30	0	0.37	0	0.3	200	0.06	0	0.3	200	0.20	0
pr136	96772	10.88	0	1.00	0	0.3	200	0.06	0	0.2	50	0.40	0
pr144	58537	6.95	0	2.18	0	0.1	200	0.25	0	0.2	50	0.08	0
pr152	73682	4.05	0	3.88	0	0.07	50	0.12	0	0.2	20	0.07	0
pr226	80369	19.89	0	11.60	0.11	0.05	200	1.00	0	0.02	250	0.66	0
pr264	49135	34.77	0	4.60	0	0.3	100	6.40	0	0.2	20	3.00	0
pr299	48191	13.92	0	3.50	0	0.25	200	1.70	0	0.2	200	1.88	0
pr439	107217	30.00	0.14	66.00	0.01	0.2	200	35.00	0	0.35	400	12.00	0
pr1002	259045	106.00	0.19	119.00	0	0.25	3000	84.00	0	0.2	700	148.00	0
pr2392	378032	0.05	0	0.05	0	0.2	200	0.05	0	0.2	200	0.05	0
rat99	1211	0.14	0.25	0.29	0	0.2	200	0.12	0	0.3	250	0.09	0
rat195	2323	7.99	0	2.38	0	0.25	50	0.60	0	0.3	250	0.18	0
rat575	6773	34.86	0.13	41.00	0.01	0.05	200	7.00	0.05	0.3	250	12.88	0
rat783	8806	15.00	0.70	339.00	0	0.1	2000	13.80	0	0.25	500	8.87	0
r11304	252948	150.00	0.08	207.00	0.34	0.1	200	345.00	0	0.4	200	200.00	0
r11323	270199	2500.00	0.12	160.00	0.05	0.2	500	341.00	0	0.2	5000	555.00	0
st70	675	1.70	0	0.48	0	0.2	200	0.06	0	0.2	200	0.08	0
ts225	126643	4.00	0	0.50	0	0.25	20	0.20	0	0.25	20	1.08	0
u159	42080	4.20	0	0.20	0	0.2	200	0.06	0	0.2	200	0.08	0

Table 2.1. (Continued)

Problem	Optimal	Self-tuning				Optimized parameters GLS-SM							
		GLS		GLS-SM		No 2-opt in initial solution				2-opt in initial solution			
		CPU	%	CPU	%	α	c^1_{max}	CPU	%	α	c^1_{max}	CPU	%
u2319	234256	1045.00	0	323.00	0.01	0.3	2500	182.00	0.01	0.35	1000	652.00	0
vm1084	239297	108.00	0.12	36.00	0.05	0.2	2000	52.00	0	0.05	500	225.00	0
vm1748	336556	180.00	0.12	547.00	0.09	0.25	5000	1272.00	0.03	0.25	5000	910.00	0
Average		106.14	0.05	47.63	0.02			60.72	0.003			70.96	0.00

2.3.3. Results for Standard TSP Benchmarks

In this section we present a comparative analysis of the results obtained with our algorithm with two state-of-art algorithms from the literature, namely version 1.1 of the Concorde cutting plane (Chvatal *et al.*, 1999) and Concorde LandK (Applegate *et al.*, 2003; Fisher and Merz, 2004). In our experiments the original implementations of both algorithms (with default parameter settings) were tested on the same computer as the GLS-SM. Because both Concorde algorithms are implemented with C++ and the GLS-SM in Visual Basic (which always results in slower computation times compared to C++ implementation), a direct comparison of CPU times is difficult.

In Table 2.2 the tested algorithms are first listed, then the number of optimal solutions obtained with the algorithm and average percentual difference of the results with respect to the optimal solutions, based on single test run. Finally, the average CPU time in seconds and the number of optimization parameters related to each algorithm are described.

Table 2.2. Comparison of results for the 43 TSP benchmarks from Table 2.1

Algorithm	NS	AI	ACPU	n
Concorde *Cutting Plane*	43	0	416.05	1
Concorde LandK	18	0.61	0.80	17
GLS-SM	43	0	70.95	2
GLS-SM Auto	33	0.018	47.62	3
GLS Auto	33	0.051	115.25	2

NS – Number of optimal solutions, AI – Average inaccuracy (%), ACPU – Average
CPU time (sec), n – number of adjusted parameters.

Based on Table 2.2, only Concorde cutting plane and the suggested GLS-SM with optimized parameters found the optimal solution to all problems. However, the CPU time of Concorde appears to be significantly (six times) higher. Concorde LandK is clearly the fastest but comes at a price, producing lower quality solutions and requiring a detailed tuning of 17 parameters. To obtain higher quality solutions with Concorde LandK, more test runs would be required, given the random nature of the algorithm. In general it appears that the suggested metaheuristic is competitive with Concorde software both in terms of computation time and solution quality.

3. MULTILOCUS GENETIC MAPPING

3.1. INTRODUCTION

This chapter is devoted to genetic mapping, i.e. one-dimensional ordering along chromosomes such elements as genes and various types of DNA markers. With n such elements, the number of all possible orders will be $n!/2$ out of which only one order is considered as the true one, representing the organization of the real chromosome. As we noted in chapter 1, the MGM is TSP-like UWSP because all ordered elements are placed on one coordinate axis only.

One of the possibilities in addressing this problem is to recover the marker order from a known matrix d_{ij} of pairwise marker distances. The special case of the problem can contain the restriction on the sequence of some (anchor) markers. Revealing the "true" marker order requires solving the UWSP with high precision and within a reasonable CPU time (Mester *et al.*, 2003a, b) since even a small change of the optimization criterion (e.g., total map length) may result in a different order of the markers. These requirements are further complicated by necessity of applying computing-intensive methods for testing the reliability of the constructed map based on the estimates of local stability of marker neighborhoods. For example, one may use bootstrap or jackknife re-sampling methods (Efron, 1979, 1993; Wang *et al.*, 1994; Liu, 1998) that suppose repeatedly solving the problem (e.g., 100-1000 times) in order to verify the obtained multilocus order (Mester *et al.*, 2003a).

In this chapter we demonstrate the application of a highly effective metaheuristic referred to as Guided Evolution Strategies (GES), to multipoint genetic mapping problems. GES combines the strengths of Guided Local

Search (Voudouris, 1997) and Evolution Strategy (Mester *et al.*, 2003a). It was successfully applied to a more complex combinatorial problem, the so-called Vehicle Routing Problems (Mester and Bräysy, 2005; Mester *et al.*, 2007). The proposed metaheuristic proved efficient and very competitive in comparison to the previous heuristic methods providing best-known solutions to 86% of 300 standard VRPTW benchmarks (see site www.top.sintef.no/vrp/benchmarks.html). In sections below we represent the particularities of adaptation of GES algorithm to MGM. For this case of TSP (UWSP) some new meta-heuristics and evolution strategies were developed (Mester *et al.*, 2003a, 2005).

3.2. EVOLUTION STRATEGIES FOR COMBINATORIAL OPTIMIZATION PROBLEMS

ES is a heuristic algorithm mimicking natural population processes. The numerical procedures in such an optimization are based on simulation of *mutation*, followed by selection of the fittest "genotypes" founded on obtained values of the optimization criterion. In contrast to GA, ES does not employ sexual process, i.e., recombination (or crossover). Various approaches were proposed for choosing the *population* size and *selection* type in the ES including the (1+1)-strategy (Rechenberg, 1973) and (μ,λ)-strategy (Schwefel, 1977). Clearly, combinatorial problems cannot be directly represented in terms of ES with real-value formulation. Combinatorial versions of ES differ from the real-value formulation by a specific representation of the solution vector x and the mutation mechanisms. Homberger and Gehring (1999) and Mester *et al.*, (2003a) adopted (μ,λ)-ES and (1+1)-ES algorithms, respectively, and proposed the combinatorial formulations for solving the vehicle routing problem with time window restrictions that is similar to multipoint analysis of markers belonging to several chromosomes (linkage groups).

In combinatorial formulation, the solution of the TSP and the UWSP can be represented as a vector $x=(x_1, x_2,..., x_n)$ that consists of n ranked discrete coordinates. At generation k, the *mutation* operator (referred to hereafter as *mutator*) changes the order of some components of vector x^k thereby producing a new solution vector x^{k+1}. The fitness function assigns to each arc (a_i, a_j) or pair of coordinates (x_i, x_j) of the solution vector x^{k+1} a non-negative d_{ij} cost of moving from element i to element j. For optimization of a combinatorial problem, one needs to define such an order of the vector coordinates (or nodes) that will provide minimum total cost $f(x)$. If after the current *selection* step $f(x^{k+1})$ is better than $f(x^k)$, then the optimization process will continue with the new solution vector x^{k+1}.

The central question in ES algorithms is about *Mutation Strategies.* Contrary to GA, mutation is the only way to change a solution in an ES algorithm. Three components of mutation strategy have to be defined for an ES algorithm. *First* component mimics the mechanism of mutation. For that, one can use *move-generation* and *solution-generation* mechanisms (Osman, 1993). The *move-generation* mechanism can be effectively applied only to a TSP where no constrains are imposed on the variables. For constrained problems, the *solution–generation* mechanisms working based on the "remove-insert" scheme (Shaw, 1998; Homberger and Gehring, 1999; Mester *et al.*, 2003a) are usually applied. The basic idea of *solution–generation* is to remove a selected set of components from current solution, and then reinsert the removed components at optimal cost. Different ways to utilize this approach are reviewed by Bräysy and Gendreau (2001a). The *second* component forms the neighborhood for mutation. Optimal size of the neighborhood is very important for solving large-scale problems. Local search on large neighborhoods (LNS) increases the CPU time. Perturbation with small neighborhoods (SN) accelerates the optimization process but can not allow to reach remote points on a large solution vector. The Variable Neighborhood strategy (VN) of Mester *et al.*, (2003a, 2007) combines the ideas of both approaches (LNS and SN), and for the large-scale problems the solution vector is divided into some specific parts (the set V of VN). The *third* component defines the size of mutation on the selected neighborhood. This is *remove* step in the "remove-insert" mutation mechanism.

In ES algorithms, usually small mutation disturbances to the solution vector are desirable. We found no clear formulation of the notion *small mutation* in the earlier literature on ES algorithms. Consequently, we attempted to provide such a formulation together with a notion of *Variable Mutation Size* (VMS) (see Mester *et al.*, 2003a). The number of removed points β is determined by $\beta = (0.2 + 0.5\xi)n^2$. Here n is the number of customers in the VN and ξ is a random value uniformly distributed between 0 and 1. The formula means that smaller VMS are used more often than intermediate and high VMS (close to $0.2+0.5*1=0.7$). Additionally, a large VMS size (i.e., $\beta=n$) is used with small probability (0.01).

3.3. THE EVOLUTION STRATEGY ALGORITHM WITH MULTI-PARAMETRIC MUTATOR (ES-MPM)

The quality of ES algorithms depends on how efficient will be the contribution of the mutation process to diversity of solutions subjected to selection. The ES algorithm described by Mester *et al.*, (2003a, b), was intended to solve moderate scale UWSP with up to 200-300 points. For this algorithm we developed the multi-parametric mutator (MPM) based on three components of the mutation strategy $M\{V, \alpha, \beta\}$, where V is a set of VN that is formed via division of the data set into special subsets; α is a parameter of the insertion operation in the "remove-insert" mutation mechanism (Mester *et al.*, 2003a), and β is a parameter of mutation size. To accelerate solving of such problems, the large-scale UWSP is divided on 8 specific parts (see Figure 3.1) and the optimization process is carried out consequently on each VN in V, so that the largest VN (numbered as v_8 in the set V) is employed with frequency 1/8 only. After successful mutation of the specific subset, MPM adaptively repeats the new mutation on current VN with another parameter β.

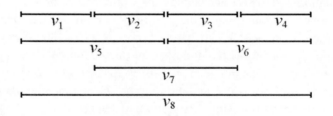

Figure 3.1. Forming set of the Variable Neighborhoods V{ v1... v8} in ES-MPM algorithm for large-scale UWSP problems.

To generate new mutated solutions, the ES algorithm removes β random components from current solution vector and reinserts these by the *best insertion* criterion with α parameter, i.e., each rejected component k will be inserted between components i and $j=i+1$, beginning from the first component of the set, while $(d_{ik}+d_{kj}-d_{ij}.) > \alpha(d_{i+1,k}+d_{k,j+1}-d_{i+1,j+1})$. Varying the value of inserting parameter α within some range (say, from 0.6 to 1.4), and with some increment (e.g., 0.2 units), we can obtain some new solutions. Three well-known improving heuristics are applied to each new solution: Reinsert (see survey Bräysy and Gendreau, 2001b), 1-interchange (Osman, 1993), and 2-opt

(Lin and Kernighan, 1973). In our algorithm, these three procedures, merged into a subroutine called *Simple Local Search* (SLS), are repeated in a loop until the current solution is improved. The best solution (out of these new ones and the last best) is selected as *current best solution* so far, and mutation process is continued in the same manner.

High efficiency of the ES approach in solving one-dimensional multilocus ordering problems (of about 50-300 markers) was demonstrated (Mester *et al.*, 2003a, b). However, the size of the real world ordering problems could be significantly larger (up 1000 or more markers per chromosome with a consequent nonlinear increase in CPU).

3.4. GUIDED EVOLUTION STRATEGIES (GES) FOR MGM

In chapter 2, we noted that both GLS and ES meta-heuristics are powerful and competitive in solving combinatorial problems. However, we clearly understand that each of these approaches is a heuristic and there is no guarantee to reach the exact solution. With such point of view, we suppose that hybrid algorithms that combine powerful properties of some metaheuristics will work somewhat better than each of them taken separately. Our successful experiments with more complicated combinatorial problems, both VRP and VRPTW (Mester and Bräysy, 2005), confirmed usefulness of the idea to combine positive properties of both algorithms (GLS and ES-MPM) in one hybrid scheme (Mester and Bräysy, 2005). In this section we describe same hybrid (GES) algorithm that was adapted for UWSP-based genomic applications. GES algorithm works in two phases. In the first phase, an initial solution is created by 2-opt local search of Lin and Kernighan (1973) whereas in the second phase an attempt is made to improve the initial solution by GES algorithm. In this hybrid algorithm, GLS is a memory-based heuristic that punishes "bad" arcs (longest and often visited in local optima) of the solution vector and forms the *Penalty Variable Neighborhood* (PVN) as a mutation region for optimization by the ES-MPM algorithm. In the GES, we define the PVN as γ random components in the vicinity of a penalty arc: $\gamma=(0.1+0.6\xi^2)n$, where $0 \leq \xi \leq 1$ is a random value, and $n=|x^k|$. In our algorithm, a large PVN ($\gamma=n$) is applied with probability 0.01. GLS generates small PVN values more often, accelerating thereby the optimization process.

The GLS and ES steps are repeated iteratively in GES, one after another, until a stopping criterion was achieved (e.g., limit of the executing time; the time during which the best solution achieved so far has not been improved, and others). More precisely, the ES algorithm is switched on if GLS cannot improve the solution during a predetermined time interval. Each ES step produces six mutations (with different inserting parameter α), and after each mutation a new constructed solution vector is improved by the SLS. Moreover, the ES steps are repeated after the successful mutations. Since the GLS step is 20-30 fold faster than the ES step, GLS runs while the counter of unsuccessful iterations (trials) b is less than a factor b_{max} predefined by the user, or the size of the current PVN is greater than some limit number (say, 200 points). Parameter b_{max} determines the ratio between the number of GLS steps and the number of ES steps in optimization process. With large b_{max} (range 25-100), the number of generated GLS solutions is also large whereas with small b_{max} (5-25) ES participates more frequently and the resulting solutions may be of higher quality. A short schema of the GES algorithm in pseudo code is represented bellow:

Phase I
Create initial solution S^0; $k = 1$; $S^k = S^0$.
         Define $b_{max} = 5 \div 100$; $b = 0$.
         Initiate penalty parameters $L = \lambda\, S^k/n$ (where $\lambda = 0.05 \div 0.3$).
         $p_i=0$ for each penalty counter.
         $S^{**}=S^0$.

Phase II
1.   GLS steps:
    Do

       1.1   Define penalty arc $a_{i,i+1}$ on current S^k by maximum $util_i$.
       1.2   Correct penalty distance matrix $(d_{i,i+1} = d_{i,i+1} + L)$ and penalty counter $(p_i=p_i+1)$.
       1.3   Define current PVN^k around the penalty arc.
       1.4   Produce 2-Opt Local Search on augmented objective function $h(PVN^k) \rightarrow S^*$.
       1.5   If $g(S^*) < g(S^{**})$ Then $b = 0$; $S^{**}=S^*$ Else $b = b + 1$.
       1.6 $k = k + 1$; $S^k = S^*$.
    Loop While $b < b_{max}$ OR size of $PVN^k > 200$.

2.   ES-MPM steps:
    Do

    2.1. Success=0

    2.2. For α =0.6 to 1.4 with step 0.2 Do.

        {

        2.3. Produce mutation M(PVN^k, α , β).

        2.4. Produce the SLS on augmented objective function $h(\text{PVN}^k) \rightarrow S^*$.

        2.5. Select best from S^* and S^{**}:

               If $g(S^*) < g(S^{**})$ Then $S^{**} = S^*$; success=1.

    }

Loop While success=1

    2.6. $b = 0$; $k=k+1$.

3.   If not terminated Then Goto step 1.1.

4.   Output S^{**}.

3.5. EXPERIMENTS ON MGM USING SIMULATED DATASETS

For experiments with TSP, researchers usually try standard problems from the internet library "TSP benchmarks" (Moscato, 1996). Standard UWSP benchmarks for genomic problems are absent in the literature, thus we simulated for our computation experiments different examples with various complications and different level of signal/noise ratio. The simulation algorithm repeatedly generated a single-chromosome mapping population F_2 for a given number of markers with dominant and codominant markers, marker misclassification, negative and positive interference, and missing data, as in our previous study of ES-based algorithms (Mester *et al.*, 2003a, b), but with a several-fold increase of the problem size (e.g., 800÷1000 markers per chromosome instead of 50÷200). In order to compare different situations, a coefficient of restoration quality $K_r=(n\text{-}1)/\sum|x_i\text{-}x_{i+1}|$ was employed, where x_i is the digit code of the *i*-th marker in the currently ordered marker sequence.

Table 3.1 represents classification of the simulated UWSPs based on three factors that complicate multilocus ordering and the reached K_r level. Clearly, the "true" marker ordering on the simulated data have $K_r = 1.0$. All experiments were produced on a processor Pentium-IV (2000 Mhz, RAM 1GB) and operation system Windows-2003XP. The software for our GES and ES-MPM algorithms was written in Visual Basic 6.0.

Table 3.1. Classification of the simulated UWSP

Class of problem	Restoring factor K_r	Complication type, %		
		MC	I	MD
E – easy	0.95-1.0	<5	<5	<5
M – middle	0.85-0.95	5-15	5-15	10-30
D – difficult	< 0.85	>15	>15	>30

MC - misclassification, I - Interference, MD - Missing data.

For a comparison of efficiency of the three algorithms (GLS, ES-MPM, and GES) on the multipoint genetic mapping problem, five classes of UWSP were simulated (with 50÷800 loci). The characteristics of performance of the algorithms are compared in Table 3.2. During the experiments, for each algorithm we registered the best (min), the worse (max), and the average (aver) CPU time to reach the optimal solution. These parameters were obtained using 100 random runs for each problem. Before each run, the components of the generated vector (x^k) were carefully reshuffled. Thus, we started with arbitrary initial points in each run. In this benchmark, all tested algorithms proved to be very fast and rather similar on problems with 50÷200 loci, but GES was the leader on difficult large-scale problems (D-400 and D-800).

Some notes about stopping (termination) criteria of the optimization process are needed. Usually, in algorithms based on mimicking natural processes (e.g., GA and ES or their hybrids GES, GGA, GTS) a stopping rule is required. Thus, the user needs to terminate the optimization process by a predetermined time or by a certain condition on the value of the goal function. This fact is especially important if one has to use such algorithms not only in getting the solution, but also in verification of the solution based on resampling procedures such as jackknife and bootstrap (e.g., Mester *et al.*, 2003a, b). One of the ways to deal with this problem is by conducting preliminary tests in order to get a reasonable empirical stopping rule. Using this approach, we defined the termination factor for the GES algorithm in resampling-based verification process for multilocus genetic mapping (see last row in Table 3.2.). For example, a 100-cycle bootstrap or jackknife verification on D-800 UWSP with time limit 350 seconds requires nearly 10 hours, and it is still a reasonable CPU time for a problem of this size. In fact, even a seven-fold reduction of the time limit gives very good results (see average CPU in Table 3.2.). Simpler algorithms (e.g., 2-Opt) require less CPU time, and should be applied for very large TSP (up 5,000-1,000,000 points) arising in technical engineering (Codenotty *et al.*, 1996). However, for genomic problems, obtaining high quality solution is by far more important than economy in CPU time. This requirement is explained by small differences in the objective function even for very dissimilar multilocus orders. For example, in the D-800 problem, 2-Opt simple local search produced a solution with minimal total length $L=619780$ with restoring coefficient $K_r=0.464$. Application of the GES gave a slightly better solution $L=619560$, with an improvement in L of only 0.03%, but the quality of ordering was significantly better: $K_r=0.859$ (improvement of 85%).

Table 3.2. Comparison performance of GLS[1], ES-MPM and GES algorithms on the five simulated UWSP classes

CPU Case	Algorithm	CPU (sec)				
		M-50	M-100	M-200	D-400	D-800
Min	GLS	-	-	0.10	6	36
	ES-MPM	-	-	0.10	18	58
	GES	-	-	0.10	4	13
Max	GLS	-	0.1	0.60	200	418
	ES-MPM	-	0.1	0.90	350	500
	GES	-	0.1	0.70	40	113
Mean	GLS	-	0.05	0.29	83	205
	ES-MPM	-	0.05	0.31	112	185
	GES	-	0.05	0.26	25	49
T_r		0.1	0.3	2.0	120	350

1) It is GES program in which ES-MPM was switched off.
Symbol "-" denotes that the CPU time was less than 0.05 sec (minimum decision of the standard system timer in the program). Mean is the average of 100 trials. T_r – recommended termination factor for GES (sec).

We conducted special experiments to analyze the effect of the neighborhood size (i.e., the size of mutations) on the rate and quality of optimization. It appeared that applying a large neighborhood (PLN) increases the executing time 5-20 fold and even more compared to PVN strategy; with a small neighborhood (PSN) an increase in the rate is overweighed by a reduced quality of the solution compared to PVN. Our approach of adaptive mutation strategy (PVN) ensures both low CPU time and high quality solutions, by using both PLN and PSN (PSN being used more frequently). Typical dependencies of the solution quality on the neighborhood size are shown in Figure 3.2.

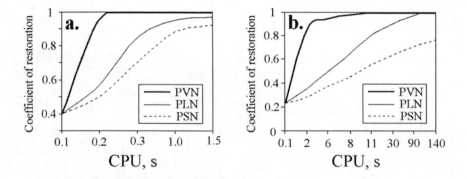

Figure 3.2. Influence of the neighborhood size of GES solutions on E-200 (a) and M-400 (b) UWSP.

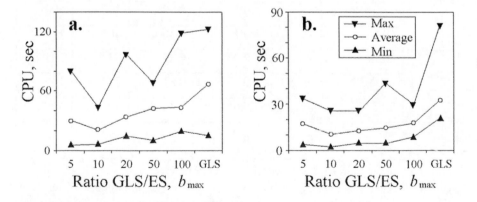

Figure 3.3. Influence of the ratio parameter bmax on the CPU time for two simulated UWSP. (a)M-800, (b) M-400.

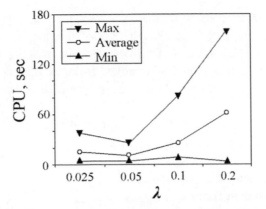

Figure 3.4. Influence of the λ (lambda) parameter on the CPU time of M-400 simulated UWSP.

Optimization process in GES algorithm is controlled by ratio parameter b_{max} and by penalty parameter λ. Typical dependence of CPU time (average, minimal, and maximal) on these parameters is shown in Figure 3.3 and 3.4. In Figure 3.3 the last value corresponds to GLS case (when ES algorithm is turned off in GES). As one can see, GES algorithm was three-fold faster than GLS with all tested ratio values. According to our experiments, the optimal values of the parameters under discussion were $b_{max}=10$ and $\lambda=0.05$.

3.6. AN APPROACH TO INCREASE THE MAP RELIABILITY BY USING VERIFICATION PROCESS

The objective of the verification procedure is detecting unstable neighborhoods in the constructed map. This can be achieved by a *jackknife* procedure (Efron, 1979): repeated re-sampling of the initial data set, e.g., using each time a certain proportion (say, 80%) of randomly chosen genotypes of the mapping population and building a new map on each such sub-sample. The identification of unstable regions can be conducted based on the frequency distribution of the right-side and left-side neighbors for each marker. The higher the deviation from 1 (i.e., from "diagonal" pattern) the less certain is local order (Figure 3.5a, b). Clearly, the unstable neighborhoods result from fluctuations of estimates of recombination rates across the repeated samples; the range of fluctuations depends on the sample size and the proportion of genotypes sampled at each jackknife run. In fact, this analysis is a modeling tool to quantify the diversity of map versions for the treated chromosome representing the sampling (stochastic) nature of the map. The results of such evaluation can be visualized to facilitate decision making about candidate problematic markers that should be removed from the map with following re-building of the map. Algorithm of this process is presented below:

1. Define distance matrix $d(i, j) = F$ (population size).
2. Build the map S_i via a TSP algorithm.
3. Accumulate the solutions S_i.
4. Jackknife on the population dataset.
5. If $i < 100$ then goto 1.
6. Detect and remove marker(s) causing local map instability.
7. If a marker was deleted then goto 2.

Figure 3.5a demonstrates a part of the map for the simulated data that contains some unstable areas. After removing three "bad" markers (numbers 6, 7 and 8) we got a map (Figure 3.5b) with stable marker ordering.

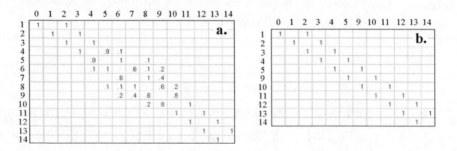

Figure 3.5 A fragment of the jackknife-based grid table for the map build on simulated data. (a) Initial order with unstable neighborhoods; (b) Stabilization of the order after removing problematic markers (# 6, 7 and 8).

4. MULTILOCUS CONSENSUS GENETIC MAPPING: FORMULATION, MODEL AND ALGORITHMS

4.1. INTRODUCTION

Numerous mapping projects conducted on various organisms have generated an abundance of mapping data. Consequently, many multilocus maps were constructed using diverse mapping populations and marker sets for the same species. The quality of maps varies broadly between studies that are based on different populations, marker sets, and used software. As one would expect, there might be some inconstancies between different versions of the maps for the same species. This proved to be the case for many organisms calling for efforts to integrate the mapping information and generate consensus maps (Klein *et al.*, 2000; Menotti-Raymond *et al.*, 2003). Recently we proposed formulations, mathematical models, and algorithms for some multilocus consensus genetic mapping (MCGM) problems (Mester *et al.*, 2005; Korol *et al.*, 2009). The main aspect of MCGM approach is requirement of identical order of shared markers for any set and subset of mapping populations. The problem of consensus mapping is even more challenging compared to multilocus mapping based on one data set, due to additional complications: differences in recombination rate and distribution along chromosomes; variations in dominance of the employed markers; different subsets of markers used by different labs. As a result, there is a clear need for being able to handle arbitrary patterns of shared sets of markers. Various formulations of MCGM problems can be considered:

a) *Multilocus genetic maps with "dominance" complication*: When building genetic maps using F_2 or F_3 data with dominant markers in the repulsion phase, we split the marker set into two groups, each with dominant markers in coupling phase only and the shared codominant markers (Peng *et al.*, 2000). Multilocus maps are then ordered for the two sets with a requirement that shared (codominant) markers should have identical order (Mester *et al.*, 2003b).

b) *Multilocus genetic maps with sex-dependent recombination:* These maps are built on the basis of male and female recombination rates represented as sex-specific matrices. Sex-specificity of the "distance" matrix may force an optimization algorithm to produce different marker orders (maps). Thus, our goal is to find the optimal solution with the restriction of the *same order* in two maps.

c) *Multilocus ordering in building consensus maps*: Such maps should be constructed based on re-analysis of raw recombination data generated in different genomic centers on different mapping populations. To solve this problem we developed a new version of *GES* algorithm which defines consensus order for all shared markers (Mester *et al.*, 2005: Korol *et al.*, 2009).

4.2. MAIN IDEA OF THE APPROACH TO SOLVE MCGM

As noted above, to solve MCGM we developed a two-phase algorithm that on *Phase I* performs multilocus ordering combined with iterative re-sampling based evaluation of the stability of marker orders. On *Phase II*, we consider consensus mapping as synchronized-TSP, and MCGM is solved by minimizing the criterion of weighted sum of recombination lengths along all multilocus maps.

For the next consideration of the consensus mapping, we will need some definitions. Let capital letters A, B and C denote sets of objects, while small letters be used for single objects. Let $L(A)$ denotes an order of A objects and, $l(a, L(A))$ is index number of object a in the order. Let C be a subset of A. We will say that $L(C)$ is partial order of $L(A)$ if and only if the sequences of C objects are the same in both orders. Namely, $L(C)$ is partial order of $L(A)$ if for any pair of C objects, c and c', from $l(c, L(C)) < l(c',L(C))$ follows that $l(c, L(A)) < l(c',L(A))$. We will say that $L(C)$ is a consensual order (CO) of two orders $L(A)$ and $L(B)$ if it is a partial order of maximal length. By the same way, consensual order of more than two orders may be defined as their maximal partial order. Then, we define a term consensus (CS) as consensual order of the consensual orders. According to these definitions, only a single consensus exists if at all. It includes shared objects of the consensual orders, since they have the same order in consensual orders.

In the case of genetic maps based on overlapping (shared) markers, two complementary sets can be defined: M_S - set of shared markers, presented in two or more maps (1) and M_U - set of unique markers presented in a single map:

$$M_S = \bigcup (M_i \cap M_j), \qquad\qquad (4.1)$$

where $i \neq j$; $i, j \in \{1,..., n\}$; n = the number of maps. M_S includes consensus markers (M_{CS}) and the others named from here as *conflicted* markers (M_{CF})

$$M_{CS} = M_S\text{-}M_{CF}. \qquad\qquad (4.2)$$

For a pair of maps the *degree of conflict* for a M_{CF} marker can be defined as the portion of consensual orders which do not include this marker. The degree of *conflict* for M_{CS} markers is always equal to zero, but the reverse is not necessarily true. It holds true for consensus markers, i.e. common markers, presented in all maps. In further consideration we will denote consensus orders by L_{CO}. The main idea to solve MCGM is to generate a set of possible orders of shared markers $L(M_{CS})$ and evaluate them by means of criterion of minimal total distance R on the datasets $i \in \{1,...,n\}$ (chromosomes) of the problem:

$$R = \Sigma\, k_i R_i \rightarrow \min, \qquad\qquad (4.3)$$

where k_i is coefficient of quality of the dataset i, and R_i is the map length of the dataset i. Each dataset i contains some shared markers $M_S(i) \in M_{CS}$ named as *anchors*, and some unique markers $M_U(i)$. For the proposed two-phase approach, we developed two different algorithms for the second phase, i.e., for searching the consensus solution to MCGM. The first one was named *Full Frame* (FF); it assumes using special heuristics for global discrete optimization in *synchronized-TSP* for all markers (unique, shared conflicting and non-conflicting). Our tests show that FF algorithm is effective with up to k = 10-15 data sets with total number of shared markers $n < 50$. For larger problems, we developed another algorithm, based on defining regions of local conflicts in the orders of shared markers (referred to as *Specific Conflicted*

Frames (SCF), followed by "local" multilocus consensus ordering for each such region. This approach allows solving much larger MCGM problems (e.g., $k > 20\text{-}30$ and $N > 100$) by moving along SCF. Solving MSGM via dissecting the chromosome into SCF includes defining sets of conflicted marker regions obtained on Phase I (based on non-synchronized solutions). Then, SCF are formed by analysis of all pairs of the resulting individual maps. Each SCF contains shared conflicting and non-conflicting markers, and some set-specific ("unique") markers. The remainder non-conflicting shared markers between the SCF regions are considered as "frozen" anchors during the solution process for each SCF region, i.e. only SCF markers participate in the optimization process. This approach significantly reduces CPU time and for small size of SCF ($m \leq 14\text{-}16$) exact solution can be obtained. For *Full Frame* (FF) approach, the optimal order of $M_U(i)$ markers on $M_S(i)$ is defined by heuristic GES algorithm (Mester *et al.*, 2004) adapted to work with anchor markers. Both FF and SCF algorithms are described in detail in the next sections.

4.3. FULL FRAME (FF) ALGORITHM FOR MCGM

Two-phase FF algorithm, based on synchronized GES algorithm (see Mester *et al.*, 2005), was improved in some aspects. For *Phase I*, GES algorithm described in section 3 was strengthen by three additional local search procedures: "Reinsert", "Reverse-Reinsert", and "Exchange1*1" (Bräysy and Gendreau, 2001b). These procedures were adapted for working with anchor marker constrains. As a result, acceleration of the optimization process and better accuracy of the solution were achieved.

For *Phase II*, new random *multi-parametric generator* of shared marker orders was developed, comprising the *mutation stage* of the optimization algorithm. For each generated order of shared markers the ordering of non-shared (chromosome specific) markers is determined by minimizing the criterion of weighted sum of recombination lengths along all individual multilocus maps (the *selection stage* of the optimization algorithm). For getting the exact solution for shared markers we must generate all ($n!/2$) possible orders. One of the ways to improve the mutation stage is to strengthen the procedure by making the main parameters of the process variable, analogous to natural processes where mutation and recombination may depend on environment and organism's fitness (Korol *et al.*, 1994). In our scheme, six parameters define the mutation strategy:

- size of mutation neighborhood $z = 1+0.25\,f^2$;
- random position $p1$ of the neighborhood;
- new random position $p2 \neq p1$ of the neighborhood;
- probability $s = 0.2$ of shifting (transposing) the neighborhood;
- probability $v = 0.2$ of reverse of the neighborhood;
- number of mutations $h = 1+2f^2$ on the new generation order,

where f is a random value uniformly distributed between 0 and 1. This mutation strategy generates short neighborhoods, so that small shifting values will appear more often among new generated orders of shared markers. Each time the mutation is performed under the best order that has been achieved so far, in accordance with the usual scheme of evolution strategy algorithms. The efficiency of the algorithms is affected by quality of the initial solutions.

Two parameters are used for estimating the quality of mapping during the optimization process:

- total distance T of shared markers, named *skeleton criterion* (SKC); and
- total distance R calculated according eq. 4.3 and named *primary criterion* (PRC).

SKC is accepted as one of starting points for ordering of shared markers. Minimum of SKC is defined by using GES algorithm; then during the process of PRC optimization, all current $T(L^i(M_S))$ and corresponding best $R(L^i(M_S), M_U)$ values are stored in a "learning" list. The process of accumulation of $T(L^i(M_S))$ and $R(L^i(M_S), M_U)$ pairs can be considered as a 'learning" process. The values of T_i and R_i from the list are correlated, although the extremes do not necessarily coincide (i.e., minimum of R may not correspond to the minimum of T. Computation time for defining criterion R could require from 0.1s to 10s depending on the problem size. Therefore, checking each generated order $L^i(M_S)$ that deviates considerably from the best PRC does not seem to be a good idea; thus we check only those $L^i(M_S)$ that satisfy the following condition:

$$T(L^i(M_S)) \leq q, \tag{4.4}$$

where parameter q is the threshold value of T (see Appendix for details on calculation of q). This limitation allows reducing significantly (20-100 folds) the computation time. Typical dependence form of the primary criterion on the skeleton criterion is shown in Figure 4.1. We keep sampling new orders for choosing q till synchronized GES algorithm is not stopped.

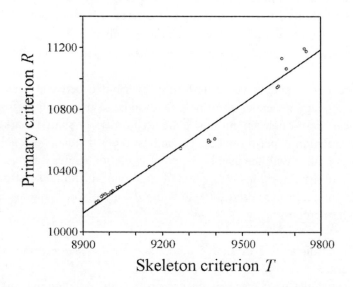

Figure 4.1 Typical dependence of the primary criterion R from the skeleton criterion T.

4.4. SPECIFIC CONFLICTED FRAMES (SCF) ALGORITHM FOR MCGM

The main idea to solve MSGM by SCF is to form sets of conflicted marker zones on the non-synchronized solutions. SCF is formed by analysis of all pairs of chromosomes. Figure 4.2 represents an example of forming SCF for a pair of chromosomes. In this example, three SCFs were formed by conflicted markers (*mar1, *mar2, *mar3; *mar11,*mar13; and *mar40, *mar41). Each SCF contains shared conflicting and non-conflicting markers, and some unique (non-shared) markers. For other markers (between the SCF), we preserve the consensus order obtained from the non-synchronized solutions. Therefore, only SCF markers participate in the optimization process by criterion (4.3).

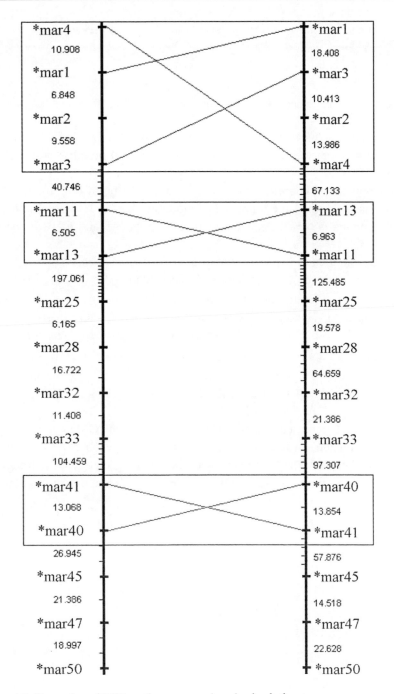

Figure 4.2. Examples of SCP on the non-synchronized solutions.

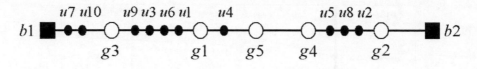

Figure 4.3. Forming order combinations of markers for SCP, where $g_i \in M_S$, $u_i \in M_U$.

This approach significantly reduces CPU time. Moreover, for small size of SCF, the problem can be solved exactly by trying all possible orders (FP) of this SCF.

Combinatorial complexity of the SCF is a function of both the number of shared markers k and the number of unique markers n. The total number of possible orders is $(n+k)!$ An example of SCF with $k=5$ and $n=10$ is shown in Figure 4.3.

The main idea of fast testing of alternative orders is based on the fact that any interval between two markers from set M_S includes a subset of markers from set M_U (in some cases this subset may be an empty set). The revealed optimal order of markers from M_U will be optimal for any interval [$b1$, $b2$] from M_S. In other words, the proposed *accelerated perturbation* (AP) algorithm prevents repeated perturbations of markers from M_U on M_S. The dependence of CPU time (in seconds) of AP and FP algorithms on n is illustrated in Table 4.1. Clearly, the advantage of AP algorithm grows with increasing n.

Table 4.2 represents consensus solution of MCGM for a simulated example with ten chromosomes and 50 markers in each chromosome; only shared markers shown. As one can see, the resulting consensus solution does not contain conflicted markers, and the ordering of shared markers is correct.

5. TSP-LIKE PROBLEM IN PHYSICAL MAPPING (PMP)

5.1. INTRODUCTION

In the last decade, genomes of many organisms were cloned in bacterial artificial chromosomes (BAC). Resulting BAC libraries can be characterized by specific markers and/or via restriction fingerprinting, resulting for each clone in a "barcode" of DNA fragments. The availability of BAC libraries with overlapping clones allows employing the barcode profiles as a tool for quantifying clone overlaps with an objective to construct physical maps (Shizuya *et al.*, 1992; Vanhouten and Mackenzie, 1999). Such maps characterize the relative positions of cloned DNA fragments in the genome and can be used in large scale DNA sequencing projects (e.g., human genome progect, Lander *et al.*, 2001; McPherson *et al.*, 2001; maize mapping project, Coe *et al.*, 2002; mouse, Gregory *et al.*, 2002), high resolution gene mapping (Faris and Gill, 2002), and map-based gene cloning (Wang *et al.*, 1995; Tanksley *et al.*, 1995). Physical mapping is long, laborious and expensive procedure, hence development of algorithms and methods making this process more effective is important, especially for dealing with large complex genomes.

One of the major steps in physical map construction is clone assembly into ordered contigs. The main idea of contig assembly it that the shared part of DNA in two clones is expected to produce shared size fragment in the fingerprint profiles of the clones. Hence, the presence of fragments (bands) with the same length in two clones c_i and c_j can indicate a possible overlap of these clones. However, the abundance of repeated elements in the genome and limited accuracy of scoring the band lengths make the data on shared bands less informative: a part of shared bands for two clones may derive from different parts of the chromosome (Soderlund *et al.*, 2000). The overlap of clones can also be tested via sequencing of clone ends and scoring the overlap of sequences. Such procedure is much more powerful but it is also much more expensive and laborious than the scoring of common bands (Venter *et al.*, 1996).

5.1.1. The Model and Problem Formulation

A chromosome can be considered as sequence of bands $(b_i)_{i\ =\ 1,...,J}$. Each band is an integer number from 1 to L. Theoretically, each clone c represents a part of this sequence: $B_c = (b_i)$, $i = i_{\text{begin}}(c),..,i_{\text{end}}(c)$. Only sets of clone bands can be observed, but not their orders and abundance within the clones. Practically, an observed band size in clone can deviate from the real one due to limited resolution of the technical system. Moreover, some of the clone bands can be missed and some extra (false) bands can be observed. Additional difficulties come from the artificial ("chimerical") clones which physically contain parts from different (non-adjacent) places of the chromosome. Using such sets of observed clone bands we need to reconstruct clone relative positions within the chromosome.

To solve this problem the clone overlaps for each pair of clones are scored as the numbers of common bands. Using theoretical distribution for clone overlaps for random clones, the statistical significance of clone overlap (p-value) can be calculated. It is expected that highly significant clone overlap corresponds to their physical overlap. Therefore, we are looking for clone orders satisfying the following requirements: (i) adjacent clones are significantly overlapping (orders with higher significances of adjacent clones are preferable); (ii) orders are long (orders containing more clones are preferable); (iii) orders are effective by overlap (i.e., order with higher sum of clone overlaps for adjacent clones are preferable). Note that some (short) clones can represent a part of genome covered by another (longer) clone. Such short clones are referred as "buried". One-dimensional ordering of a set of clones containing buried clones can be problematic (for example, in a situation of four clones c_1, c_2, c_3 and c, such as c is buried in c_2, and clones c_1 and c_3 overlap only with c_2). Nevertheless, buried clones can be considered as attached to the ordered chain of non-buried clones. Buried clones can provide additional information about relative position of bands within clones and prove clone ordering (Fasulo *et al.*, 1998).

5.1.2. Standard Methodology for Solving Physical Mapping Problem

A standard program package FingerPrinted Contigs (FPC) assembles clones into contigs by using either the end-labeled double digest method (Coulson *et al.*, 1986; Gregory *et al.*, 1997) or the complete digest method (Olson *et al.*, 1986; Marra *et al.*, 1999). Because of computational challenge of ordering huge amount of clones (about 10^4-10^5 per chromosome), FPC subdivides the set of clones on relatively small clusters of strongly overlapped clones (up to 20-50 per cluster). Clones of each cluster are ordered using local optimization and building band maps. The next step is merging the resulted orders into contigs under less restrictive conditions for clone overlaps allowing only end-to-end merging (Soderlund *et al.*, 2000). FPC uses uniform significance stringency to decide about clone overlap. To obtain relatively small cluster sizes, FPC applies very stringent level of significance; so that many pairs of clones that in fact overlap physically do not overcome this level. As a result, many singletons and short clusters appear where ordering of clones is questionable. End-to-end merging of short condigs is also problematic. Using more liberal significance stringency can lead to appearance of contigs with non-linear structure caused by problematic ("questionable", Q-) clones and by false significant overlapping.

Local optimization also can be not effective to find optimal clone order and proper band map construction: even a small error in clone ordering can lead to situations where clones "jump" from the correct position to the first vacant place. In particular, it can result in high inconsistence in clone overlaps and their positions in the resulted map of bands within the contig. If adjacent within the contig clones have non-significant number of common bands, then one can expect that these clones will show poor overlap also at the sequence level. This will lead to splitting of the contig into shorter sub-contigs.

5.1.3. An Alternative Approach to Contig Assembly

Here we present elements of our new approach to contig assembly. Alternatively to a standard FPC one, we start from clone clustering with relatively liberal overlap stringency (cutoff of significance level). Then, we conduct stepwise clustering with ever increasing stringency coordinated with assessment of the topological structure of the resulting clustering. In each cluster we order clones by using global optimization heuristics developed for solving standard TSP. Based on computing-intensive jackknife resampling analysis, we detect and exclude from the contig clones that disturb consensus clone order. This leads to appearance of well ordered contigs that can be merged into longer contigs by relaxing cutoff, under topological control of cluster structure. Our methods allow the construction of reliable and longer contigs, detection of "weak" connections in contigs and their "repair", as well as the elongation of contigs obtained by other assembly methods.

5.2. Reducing PMP to Standard TSP

Our algorithm of contig construction includes the next steps: (i) calculation of p-value for clone overlaps; (ii) grouping clones into reliable size clusters with linear topological structure; (iii) one-dimensional ordering using global optimization; (iv) re-sampling based verification of the obtained order; and (v) merging of contigs into longer contigs. In the first stage we calculate all pair-wise p-values $Pr(c_i, c_j)$ of clone overlapping and select a threshold Pr_0 (cutoff) to define clones c_i and c_j with $Pr(c_i, c_j) < Pr_0$ that can be referred to as significantly overlapping. A proper choice of the threshold Pr_0 should provide a reasonable tradeoff between two requirements: (a) to provide enough number of pairs of overlapped clones, and (b) to reduce the proportion of false overlaps among selected clone pairs.

Alternatively to the standard FPC strategy, where falsely significant clone overlaps and chimerical clones are identified by using band map in while ordering of highly significantly overlapped clones, we exclude putatively false significant overlaps and putatively chimerical clones at the stage of clustering. The excluded clones and overlaps can be used later in attempts to merge contigs. Our main idea of identification of problematic clones and clone overlaps is that each part of the chromosome is most probably covered by several clones (although in fact, some parts can be uncovered or poorly covered by clones). We expect that chimerical clones and false clone overlaps usually are not proven by parallel clones.

Clustering would subdivide clones into groups covering different parts of the chromosome. We cluster clones in such a way that a whole chromosome part (without ends), that covered by clones from the cluster, is covered by several significantly overlapped clones. Moreover, we require that, even after excluding from the consideration any single clone or clone overlap, for any pair of clones c_i and c_j from the cluster C_0 there exist a sequence of clones $c_{(1)},..,c_{(n)}$ from C_0 such as $c_{(1)}=c_i$, $c_{(n)}=c_j$ and overlap of clones $c_{(k)}$ and $c_{(k+1)}$ is significant for all $k=1,..,n-1$. For clones from such clusters we define distance based on p-value of clone overlaps to be equal to infinity for non-significantly overlapped clones (see below). After excluding buried clones, the problem of clone ordering is reduced to the standard TSP problem without requiring return to the initial point.

5.2.1. Clustering Algorithm

Let Pr_0 be a liberal level of cutoff (we used $10^{-3}/N^2$, where $N\sim10^4$-10^6 is the number of clones in a physical mapping project). With calculating all pair-wise clone overlaps Pr we subdivide the clone database into clusters by single-linkage algorithm (Jain and Dubes, 1988). Ordering of clusters with large number of clones is a computationally challenging problem. This is why stringent cutoffs are usually used to subdivide large clusters into small-to-intermediate ones. FPC uses uniform cutoff for entire database to decide if a pair of clones belong to one cluster in single-linkage clustering algorithm. However, database can contain cluster(s) with a very large number of highly significantly overlapped clones. In such situation, applying uniform cutoff may result in a solution with a few very big clusters and a lot of extremely small clusters. Further dividing of the big clusters leads to the appearance of numerous very small clusters reducing the chance of getting large contigs. Instead of uniform cutoff we propose a procedure with adaptively increasing cutoff stringency (say by three orders of magnitude).

We start clustering with a liberal cutoff Pr_0, and select the resulting reasonable size (rs) clusters, say clusters with size up to 300 clones. For each cutoff level we consider each cluster of clones as a *net* of significant overlaps (where net vertices correspond to clones and edges correspond to significant relative to Pr_0 clone overlaps). In this net we identify and temporally exclude from the analysis clones and clone overlaps not proven by parallel paths (see Figure 5.1a). For convenience, we refer to such procedure as TENPP-procedure with a respective cutoff Pr_θ. After TENPP-procedure we run single linkage algorithm on large clusters. At the next step, we increase the stringency, but only after removing from the consideration the selected reasonable size clusters (i.e., protecting them from further "dissolving"). After running this algorithm, rs-clusters are again considered as a net of significant overlaps and is subdivided into sub-clusters such as corresponding net is subdivided into parts having linear topological structure (see Figure 5.1b and paragraph 5.2.2. below). The scheme of our clustering algorithm is illustrated in Figure 5.2.

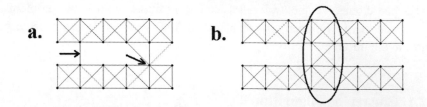

Figure 5.1 Splitting clones into clusters with linear topological structure. Set of significant clone overlaps considered as net: vertices correspond to clones, pair of vertices connected by edge if overlap of respective clones is significant. (a) Excluding of clones and clone overlaps not proven by short (of 2-4 edges) parallel paths. First we detect and exclude from the analysis non-proven clone overlaps, and only after this we detect and exclude non-proven clones. Excluded edges and vertices in the presented example are marked by arrows. (b) Excluding clones in branching. In the presented example set of such clones is marked by ellipse. Remained set of clones is subdivided into four clusters having linear topological structure by standard single-linkage algorithm.

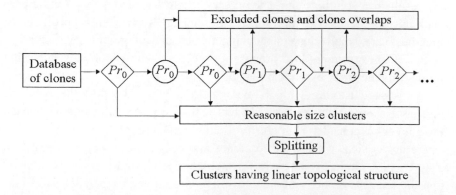

Figure 5.2 Scheme of clone clustering with adapting cutoff. Diamonds denote single-linkage clustering with corresponding cutoff. Circles denote procedure of excluding from the analysis clones and clone overlaps not proven by parallel paths in the net of significant (relative to corresponding cutoff) clone overlaps.

5.2.2. Looking for Linear Topological Structure

Although after TENPP procedure any non-excluded significant clone overlap has a parallel path (may pass through temporally excluded clones), some of the overlaps still can be false significant and some of the non-excluded clones can be chimerical. Such overlaps and chimeras can lead to situations where cluster of clones represented in the form of a net of significant overlaps will have non-linear topological structure (Figure 5.1b) incompatible with one-dimensional structure of eukaryotic chromosome. Clearly, ordering such clusters is problematic. To overcome this problem, we propose to split clusters into sub-clusters having linear topological structure by excluding from the analysis clones at the branching nodes (Figure 5.1b). Non-linearity of cluster structure can be detected by scoring ranks of vertices relative to some diametric path (any of possible diametric paths can be employed). Remind that, by definition, diametric path is the longest, in sense of number of edges, non-reducible path (e.g., Bollobas, 2002). The presence of vertices with not too small ranks (e.g., more than 2) points to non-short offshoots from the selected diametric path and, hence, a possibility of non-linear structure. Maximal rank can depend on selection of diametric path (up to twice). Hence formulated criterion for non-linearity detection is sufficient but not necessary. Clones and overlaps causing non-linearity are excluded from the analysis only at the stage of sub-contig ordering, although some of them may be used later for merging of sub-contigs into a contig.

5.2.3. Multipoint Ordering Using Global Optimization

As it was mentioned above, we propose ordering the clusters proved to have linear topological structure based on statistical significance of clone overlaps. We formulate the ordering problem in terms of global maximization of some criterion (similar to Fickett and Cinkosky, 1992; Alizadah *et al.*, 1993; Ben-Dor and Chor, 1997; Flibotte *et al.*, 2004). For simplicity, we consider only the situation where all clones are not buried. Such situation can be achieved by temporal excluding of buried clones from the analysis, although sometime it can lead to loosing the contig connectedness. The criterion $W(\Omega)$ of clone order $\Omega=(c_{\Omega(1)},\ldots, c_{\Omega(n)})$ is calculated as:

$$W(\Omega) = \sum_{i=1,\ldots,n-1} W_i(\Omega) - b(\Omega)W_0 = \sum -\log Pr(c_{\Omega(i)}, c_{\Omega(i+1)}) - b(\Omega)W_0, \quad (5.1)$$

where $b(\Omega)$ is the number of adjacent (within order Ω) clones with $Pr(c_{\Omega(i)},$ $c_{\Omega(i+1)})$>Pr_0 and W_0 is the penalty for non-significant overlapping of adjacent clones.

Maximization of such criterion can be reformulated as standard TSP without requiring of return to the starting point. Let W_{max} be the maximum of -log $Pr(c_i, c_j)$. We define distance between two clones as

$$d(c_i, c_j) = W_{max}\text{-}(\text{-log } Pr(c_i, c_j))+W_0 \ \mathbf{1}\{Pr(c_i, c_j) > Pr_0\}, \qquad (5.2)$$

where $1\{Pr(c_i, c_j) > Pr_0\}$ is indicator function equal to 1, if $Pr(c_i, c_j) > Pr_0$, and equal to zero otherwise. Global optimization is especially effective if additional information on DNA markers is also available (Flibotte *et al.*, 2004). Solution of TSP is considered as NP-hard problem. Nevertheless, good heuristics (e.g, based on evolutionary strategy optimization) for the solution of TSP were developed for situations where the number of vertices is up to order of 10^3 (Mester *et al.*, 2004).

5.2.4. Re-Sampling Verification of the Obtained Solution

The quality of ordering of clones within the contig is characterized not only by the value of the chosen criterion, but also by its robustness to small uncertainty of band content of the clones, that can be referred to as contig stability. To evaluate this stability we use jackknife iterations. Namely, we first construct the order using clone overlaps scored over all bands. In addition, we construct orders using clone overlaps based on randomly selected subsets of bands (95% of the total set). Then, the identification of unstable regions can be conducted based on the frequency distribution of the right-side and left-side neighbors for each clone in the contig order. The higher the deviation from 1 (i.e., from the "diagonal" pattern) the less certain is the local order (Mester *et al.*, 2003). One of the main reasons of appearance unstable orders is high similarity of parallel clones that may differ mainly due to noise unavoidable under any technology. Excluding of parallel clones allows constructing stable "skeleton" map, analogously to the approach suggested for building genetic maps (see section 3.6).

5.2.5. Merging of Sub-Contigs

After ordering, we try to elongate the resulted contigs by merging contigs displaying end-to-end significant overlaps (that may be also achicvablc via adding 1-2 connecting clones, or by adding singletons. First, we return to analysis all clones and clone overlaps temporally excluded at previous stages. To elongate a concrete contig we search for all clones connected (by significant overlapping or via short path of significant overlaps) with the clones from ends of the contig. If adding of all these clones (for one of the two contig ends) does not lead to violation of contig linearity, then such elongation does not seem to be problematic. If adding of these clones does leads to branching (i.e., contradicts to linear structure of the chromosome), then each of the possibilities of linear elongations (Figure 5.3) must be considered. The correct elongation can be detected by testing of clone overlapping based on clone-end sequencing (Venter *et al.*, 1996). The same problem arises if clones from one contig significantly overlap with middle clones from another contig. Availability of DNA markers (in clones) with known chromosomal position can help to reject merging of contigs from different chromosomal zones. Contigs having clones with markers from different chromosomal zones must be divided. Contigs resulting from elongation should be reordered (see section 5.2.3).

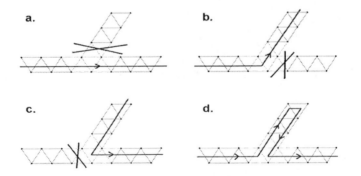

Figure 5.3 End-to-end merging of contigs. Three contigs with linear topological structure (significant clone overlaps marked by solid lines) are end-to-end connected via additional clones and significant clone overlaps (possibly excluded in previous stages, marked by doted lines). There are several possibilities of merging: (a), (b), (c) end-to-end merging of two contigs (overlaps with clones from the third contigs considered as false significant); (d) merging of all three contigs with reordering clones in the second one.

6. CONCLUSIONS

Several problems in modern genome mapping analysis belong to the field of discrete optimization on a set of all possible orders. In this paper we propose formulations, mathematical models and algorithms for genetic/genomic problem that can be formulated in TSP-like terms. These problems are considered as computationally challenging because of noisy marker scores, large-size data sets, specific constraints on certain classes of orders, and other complications. These complications do not allow to use directly both known exact and heuristic discrete optimization methods (e.g. Cutting-plane, Genetic algorithm with EAX crossover and the famous Lin-Kernighan). For solving the genome mapping problems we developed Guided Evolution Strategy heuristic based on Guided Local Search and Evolution Strategy algorithms. Both GLS and ES algorithms in GES are working together; employment of "the variable neighborhood" and multi-parametric mutation process empower the optimization algorithm.

An approach to increase the reliability of multilocus map ordering was presented here based on jackknife re-sampling as a tool for testing of the map quality. Detection and removing markers responsible for local map instabilities and non-monotonic change in recombination rates allows building stable skeleton maps with minimal total length. Further improvement of mapping quality is achievable by joint analysis of mapping data from different mapping populations. Separate ordering of different data sets does not guarantee obtaining identical orders for shared markers in resulting maps, calling for detection and removing conflicting markers. An alternative (presented above) is building de novo a consensus multilocus map based on "synchronized ordering" rather than merging the previously derived maps. This approach is also applicable in situations of gender dependent recombination and combined analysis of genetic and physical mapping data, possibly in sequential experimentation manner.

In this paper we demonstrated on the genetic and genomic TSP-like applications that proposed Guided Evolution Strategy algorithms successfully solves these constrained discrete optimization problems. The efficiency of the proposed algorithms is demonstrated on standard TSP problems and on three genetic/genomic problems with up to 2,500 points.

ACKNOWLEDGMENT

This research was partially supported by Binational Agricultural Research and Development Fund (BARD research project US-3873-06), by the Israel Ministry of Absorption, FP7-212019 research grant, and by the EDGE project funded by the Research Council of Norway and Jenny and Antti Wihuri Foundation.

APPENDIX. CHOOSING THRESHOLD Q VALUE FOR PRC CALCULATION

Let PRC and SKC be already calculated for n different orders of skeleton markers (we used $n \geq 100$). For the current SKC value, we want to decide whether the calculation of PRC (which takes much more CPU time than SKC) is desirable. As a model of relationship between SKC and PRC the following linear approximation is used:

$$R_i = R_{\text{mean}} + b(T_i - T_{\text{mean}}) + e_i,$$

where R_i and T_i are PRC and SKC values for the i-th order of skeleton markers, respectively; R_{mean} and T_{mean} are the mean values for PRC and SKC for all possible orders of skeleton markers; b is the regression coefficient; and e_i is the current difference between R_i and $R_{\text{mean}} + b(T_i - T_{\text{mean}})$.

Let p_0 be the level of significance (for example $p_0 = 5\%$), and e_0 be the quintile of p_0 level for sample distribution of e, i.e. np_0^{th} element of the ordered by increasing sequence of e_i values. Values R_{mean} and b can be estimated by least squares method. Let $R_{\text{best}} = \min_i R_i$ and T be observed SKC value for the current order of skeleton markers. To make a decision on weather PRC should be calculated, we score $R_e = R_{\text{mean}} + b(T - T_{\text{mean}})$. If the $R_e + e_0 > R_{\text{best}}$, then we suppose that PRC for such skeleton order is higher (with probability $1 - p_0$) than the obtained R_{best} and do not calculate it. Thus, $q = T_{\text{mean}} - (R_{\text{mean}} - R_{\text{best}} + e_0)/b$.

REFERENCES

Alizadah, F., Karp, R., Newberg, L. A., and Weisser, D. (1993). Physical mapping of chromosomes: A combinatorial problem in molecular biology. In *Proceedings of the Fourth Annual ACM_SIAM symposium on DiscreteAlgorithms,* pp. 371-381.

Applegate, D., Cook, W., and Rohe, A. (2003). Chained Lin-Kernighan for large traveling salesman problems. *IJOC, 15,* pp. 82-92.

Ben-Dor, A., and Chor, B. (1997). On constructing radiation hybrid maps. *Journal of Computational Biology, 4,* pp. 517-534.

Bollobas, B. (2002). *Modern Graph Theory,* (1st ed.) Springer.

Bräysy, O., and Gendreau, M. (2001a). Metaheuristics for the vehicle routing problem with time windows. Internal Report STF42 A01025, SINTEF Applied Mathematics, Department of Optimization, Norway.

Bräysy, O., and Gendreau, M. (2001b). Route construction and local search algorithm for the vehicle routing problem with time windows. Internal Report STF42 A01025, SINTEF Applied Mathematics, Department of Optimization, Norway.

Burkard, R., Deineko, V., van Dal, R., van der Veen, J., and Woeginger, G. (1998). Well-solvable special cases of the travelling salesman problem: a survey. *SIAM Rev.,* 40, pp. 496–546.

Chvatal V., Applegate, D., Bixby, R., and Cook, W. (1999). Concorde: a code for solving travelling salesman problems (http://www.math.princeton.edu/tsp/concorde.html)

Codenotty, B., Margara, L., and Resta, G. (1996). Perturbation: An efficient technique for the solution of very large instances of the Euclidean TSP. *Informs Journal on Computing, Vol. 8(2),* pp. 125-133.

Coe, E., Cone, K., McMullen, M., Chen, S., Davis, G., Gardiner, J., Liscum, E., Polacco, M., Paterson, A., Sanchez-Villeda, H., Soderlund, C., and

Wing, R. (2002). Access to the maize genome: an integrated physical and genetic map. *Plant Physiology*, *128*, pp. 9-12.

Coulson, A., Sulston, J., Brenner, S., and Kam, J. (1986). Toward a physical map of the genome of the nematode *C.elegans*. *Proc. Natl Acad. Sci. USA*, *83*, pp. 7821-7825.

Cowling, P. (1995). Optimization in steel hot rolling. In: *Optimization in industry*. Wiley, Chichester, pp. 55-66.

Cowling, P., and Keuthen, R. (2005). Embedded local search approaches for routing optimization. *Comp and Oper Res*, *32*, pp. 465–490.

Efron, B. (1979). Bootstrap method: Another look at the jackknife. *Ann. Stat.*, *7*, pp. 1-26.

Efron, B., and Tibshirani, R. (1993). *An Introduction to the Bootstrap*. Chapman and Hall, New York.

Ellis, T. (1997). Neighbour mapping as a method for ordering genetic markers. *Genet. Res. Camb.*, *69*, pp. 35-43.

Emrich, S. J., Aluru, S., Fu, Y., Wen, T. J., Narayanan, M., Guo, L., Ashlock, D. A., and Schnable, P. S. (2004). A strategy forassembling the masize(Zea mays L.) genome. *Bioinformatics*, *20*, pp. 140-147.

Falk, C. T. (1992). Preliminary ordering of multiple linked loci using pairwise linkage data. *Genetic Epidemiology*, *9*, pp. 367-375.

Faris, J. T., and Gill, B. S. (2002). Genomic targeting and high-resolution mapping of the domestication gene Q in wheat. *Genome*, *45,* pp. 706–718.

Fasulo, D., Jiang, T., Karp, R. M., and Sharma, N. (1998). Constructing maps using the span and inclusion relations. In *RECOMB. Proceedings of the Second Annual International Conference on Computational Molecular Biology*. Edited by: Istrail, S., Pevzner, P., Waterman, M., New York, NY, USA: ACM. pp. 64-73.

Fickett, J., and Cinkosky, M. (1992). A genetic algorithm for assembling chromosome physical maps. In Lim,H., Fickett,J., Cantor, C., and Robbins, R. (Eds), *The Second International Conference on Bioinformatics. Supercomputing and Complex Genomic Analysis*. World Scientific, New Jersey, pp. 273-285.

Flibotte, S. R., Chiu, R., Fjell, C., Krzywinski, M., Schein, J. E., Shin, H., and Marra, M. A. (2004). "Automated ordering of fingerprinted clones". *Bioinformatics*, *20(8)*.

Fisher, T., and Merz, P. (2004). Embedding a chained Lin-Kernighan algorithm into a distributed algorithm. Report 331/04, University of Kaiserslautern.

Flood, M. M. (1956). The travelling-salesman problem. *Oper. Res.*, *4*, pp. 61–75.

Gamboa, D., Rego, C., and Glover, F. (2006). Implementation analysis of efficient heuristic algorithms for the traveling salesman problem. *Comp. and Oper. Res.*, *33*, pp. 1154–1172.

Givry, S., Bouchez, M., Chabrier, P., Milan, D., and Schiex, T. (2001). CarthaGene: multipopulation integrated genetic and radiation hybrid mapping. *Bioinformatics*, *8*, pp. 1703-1704.

Gregory, S. G., Howell, G., and Bentley, D. (1997). Genome mapping by fluorescent fingerprinting. *Genome Res.*, *7*, pp. 1162–1168.

Gregory, S., Sekhon, M., Schein, J., *et al.*, (2002). A physical map of the mouse genome. *Nature, 418*, pp. 743–750.

Hall, D., Bhandarkar, M., Arnold, J., and Jiang, T. (2001). Physical mapping with automatic capture of hybridization data. *Bioinformatics*, *3*, 205-213.

Helsgaun, K. (2000). An effective implementation of the Lin-Kernighan traveling salesman heuristic. *Eur. J. Oper. Res.*, *1*, pp. 106–130.

Homberger, J., and Gehring, H. (1999). Two evolutionary metaheuristics for vehicle routing problem with time windows. *INFOR, 37*, pp. 297-318.

Jackson, B., Schnable, P., and Aluru, S. (2007). Consensus genetic maps as median orders from inconsistent sourses. *Transactions on Computational Biology and Bioinformatics*, in press.

Jain, A. K., and Dubes, R.C. (1988). "Algorithms for clustering data." Englewood Cliffs, N.J.: Prentice Hall.

Johnson, D., and MCGeoch, L. (2002). Experimental analysis of heuristics for the STSP. In: Gutin, G., Punnen, A. (eds) The traveling salesman problem and its variations. Kluwer, Dordrecht, pp. 369–443.

Korol, A. B., Preygel, I. A., and Preygel, S. I. (1994). *Recombination Variability and Evolution*. Chapman and Hall, London.

Korol, A., Mester, D., Frenkel, Z., and Ronin, Y. (2009). Methods for genetic analysis in the *Triticeae*. *In:* Feuillet, C., and Muehlbauer, G. (eds). *Genetics and Genomics of the Triticeae*. Springer, pp. 163-199.

Lander, E. S., Linton, L. M., Birren, B., *et al.*, (2001). Initial sequencing and analysis of the human genome. *Nature, 409*, pp. 860–921.

Lawler, E., Lenstra, J., Kan, A., and Shmoys, D. (1985). The traveling salesman problem. Wiley, New York.

Lin, S., and Kernighan, B. (1973). An effective heuristic algorithm for the TSP. *Operation Research, 21*, pp. 498-516.

Lin, K., and Chen, C. (1996). Layout-driven chaining of scan flip-flops. *IEE Proc. Comp. Dig. Tech.*, *143*, pp. 421–425.

Liu, B. H., (1998). *Statistical Genomics: Linkage, Mapping, and QTL Analysis*. CRC Press, New York.

Marra, M., Kucaba, T., Sakhon, M., *et al.*, (1999) A map for sequence analysis of the *Arabidopsis thaliana* genome. *Nat. Genet., 22*, pp. 265–275.

McPherson, J. D., Marra, M., Hillier, L., *et al.*, (2001) A physical map of the human genome. *Nature, 409*, pp. 934–941.

Mester, D., Ronin, Y., Minkov, D., Nevo, E., and Korol, A. (2003a). Constructing large scale genetic maps using evolution strategies algorithm. *Genetics, 165*, pp. 2269–2282.

Mester, D., Ronin, E., Nevo, E., and Korol, A. (2003b). Efficient multipoint mapping: making use of dominant markers repulsion-phase. *Theor Appl Genet, 107,* pp.1002–1112.

Mester, D., Korol, A., and Nevo, E. (2004). Fast and high precision algorithms for optimization in large scale genomic problems. *Comput Biol and Chem, 28*, pp. 281–290.

Mester, D., Ronin, Y., Korostishevsky, M., Picus, V., Glazman, A., and Korol, A. (2005). Multilocus consensus genetic maps: formulation, algorithms and results. *Computation Biology and Chemistry, 30*, pp. 12-20.

Mester, D., and Braysy, O. (2005). Active guided evolution strategies for large scale vehicle routing problems with time windows. *Comp. and Oper. Res., 32*, pp.1593–1614.

Mester, D., and Braysy, O. (2007). Active guided evolution strategies for large scale capacitated vehicle routing problems. *Comp. and Oper. Res., 34*, pp. 2964-2975.

Mester, D., Bräysy, O., and Dulaert, W. (2007). A multi-parametric evolution strategies algorithm for vehicle routing problems. *Expert Systems with Application, 32*, pp. 508-717.

Moscato, P. (1996). TSPBIB, Available from: URL: *http://www.densis.fee.unicamp.br/~moscato/TSPBIB_home.html*.

Mott, R. F., Grigoriev, A. V., Maier, E., Hoheisel, J. D., and Lehrach, H. (1993). Algorithms and software tools for ordering clone libraries: application to the mapping of the genome of Schizosaccharomyces pombe. *Nucleic Acids Research, 21,* pp.1965-1974.

Nagata, Y., and Kobayashi, S. (1997). Edge Assembly Crossover: A High-power Genetic Algorithm for the Traveling Salesman Problem, *Proc. of 7th Int. Conf. on Genetic Algorithms*, pp. 450-457.

Nagata, Y. (2007). Edge Assembly Crossover for the Capacitated Vehicle Routing Problem, *Proc. of 7th Int. Conf. on Evolutionary Computation in Combinatorial Optimization*, pp. 142–153.

Olson, M. V., Dutchik, J. E., Graham, M. Y., Brodeur, G. M., Helms, C., Frank, M., MacCollin, M., Scheinman, R., and Frank, T. (1986). Random-clone strategy for genomic restriction mapping in yeast. *Proc. Natl. Acad. Sci.*, *83*, pp. 7826–7830.

Olson, J. M., and Boehnke, M. (1990). Monte Carlo comparison of preliminary methods of ordering multiple genetic loci. *American Journal of Human Genetics*, *47*, pp. 470-482.

Osman, I. H. (1993). Metasrategy simulated annealing and tabu search algorithm for VRP. *Annals of Operation Research, 41*, pp. 421-451.

Ott, G. (1991). *Analysis of Human Genetic Linkage.* The John Hopkins University Press, Baltimore and London.

Papadimitiou, C., and Steiglitz, K. (1981). Combinatorial optimization: Algorithms and complexity. Prentice-Hall, Englewood Cliffs.

Pekney, J., and Miller, D. (1991). Exact solution of the no-wait flowshop scheduling problem with a comparison to heuristic methods. *Comp. and Chem. Eng., 15*, pp. 741–748.

Rechenberg, I. (1973). *Evolutionstrategie.* Fromman-Holzboog, Stuttgart.

Renaud, J., Boctor, F., and Laporte, G. (1996). Fast composite heuristic for symmetric TSP. *IJOC, 2*, pp. 134–143.

Reinelt, G. (1991). TSPLIB - a travelling salesman problem library. *ORSA J. Comput., 3,* pp. 376–384.

Reinelt, G. (1994). *The travelling salesman.* Lecture Notes in Computer Science 840. Springer, Berlin.

Schiex, T., and Gaspin, C. (1997). Carthagene: constructing and joining maximum likelihood genetic maps. *ISMB, 5*, pp. 258-267.

Shaw, P. (1998). Using constraint programming and local search methods to solve vehicle routing problems. In Maher, M., and Puget, J.-F. (eds.): *Principles and Practice of Constraint Programming – CP98, Lecture Notes in Computer Science*, Springer-Verlag, New York, pp. 417–431.

Schneider, J. (2003). Searching for Backbones – a high performance parallel algorithm for solving combinatorial optimization problems. *Fut. Gen. Comp. Syst., 19*, pp. 121–131.

Schwefel, H-P. (1977). *Numeriche optimierung von vomputer-modellen mittels der evolutions strategie.* Birkauser, Basel.

Shizuya, H., Birren, B., Kim, U. J., Mancino, V., Slepak, T., Tachiiri, Y., and Simon, M. (1992). Cloning and stable maintenance of 300-kilobase-pair fragments of human DNA in *Escherichia coli* using an F-factor–based vector. *PNAS, 89*, pp. 8794–8797.

Soderlund, C., Humphray, S., Dunham, A., and French, L. (2000). Contigs built with fingerprints, markers, and FPC V 4.7. *Genome Res.*, *10*, pp. 1772–1787.

Tanksley, S. D., Ganal, M. W., and Martin, G. B. (1995). Chromosome landing: a paradigm for map-based gene cloning in plants with large genomes. *Trends Genet.*, *11*, pp. 63–68.

Tsai, C-F., Tsai, C-W., and Tseng, C-C. (2004). A new hybrid heuristic approach for solving large traveling salesman problem. *Inf. Sciences.*, *166*, pp. 67–81,

Tsang, E., and Voudouris, C. (1997). Fast local search and guided local search and their application to British telecom's workforce scheduling problem. *Oper. Res. Let.*, *20*, pp. 119–127.

Vanhouten, W., and Mackenzie, S. (1999). Construction and characterization of a common bean bacterial artificial chromosome library. *Plant Mol. Biol.*, *40*, pp. 977-983.

Venter, J. C., Smith H. O., and Hood, L. (1996). A new strategy for genome sequencing. *Nature, 381*, pp. 364–366.

Voudouris, C. (1997). Guided local search for combinatorial problems. PhD Thesis, University of Essex, Colchester.

Walshaw, C. (2002). A multilevel approach to the travelling salesman problem. *Oper. Res.*, *50*, pp. 862–877.

Weeks, D., and Lange, K. (1987). Preliminary ranking procedures for multilocus ordering. *Genomics, 1*, pp. 236-242.

Wang, Y., Prade, R., Griffith, J., *et al.*, (1994). S_BOOTSTRAP: Assessing the statistical reliability of physical maps by bootstrap resampling. *Cabios*, *10,* pp. 625-634.

Wang, G. L., Holsten, T. E., Song, W. Y., Wang, H. P., and Ronald, P. C. (1995). Construction of a rice bacterial artificial chromosome library and identification of clones linked to the Xa-21 disease resistance locus. *Plant J., 7*, pp. 525–533.

INDEX